Complex Cases and Comorbidity in Eating Disorders

Riccardo Dalle Grave • Massimiliano Sartirana
Simona Calugi

Complex Cases and Comorbidity in Eating Disorders

Assessment and Management

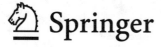 Springer

Riccardo Dalle Grave
Eating and Weight Disorders Department
Villa Garda Hospital
Garda
Verona
Italy

Massimiliano Sartirana
Adolescent and Adult Eating and Weight
Disorders Clinical Service
Associazione Disturbi Alimentari
Verona
Italy

Simona Calugi
Eating and Weight Disorders Department
Villa Garda Hospital
Garda
Verona
Italy

ISBN 978-3-030-69343-5   ISBN 978-3-030-69341-1   (eBook)
https://doi.org/10.1007/978-3-030-69341-1

This Springer imprint is published by the registered company Springer Nature Switzerland AG
The registered company address is: Gewerbestrasse 11, 6330 Cham, Switzerland

Preface

Eating disorders are almost always "complex cases", as the great majority of such patients have other significant clinical problems. Most meet the diagnostic criteria for another mental disorder and are often recipients of a diagnosis of some personality disorder. Marked interpersonal difficulties and severe psychosocial impairment are common. Moreover, physical complications are almost always present, and, in a subgroup of patients, a general medical condition coexists and interacts with the eating disorder psychopathology.

Clinicians often use the term "comorbidity" to describe the clinical problems that coexist with eating disorders. The term has become commonly used, and somewhat "fashionable" in psychiatric circles, to indicate not only those cases in which a patient is diagnosed with a psychiatric disorder and a medical one (e.g. major depression and type 2 diabetes), but also those cases in which the patient receives a diagnosis of two or more psychiatric disorders (e.g. major depression and panic disorder).

However, comorbidity is a complex issue, both conceptually and clinically. From a conceptual point of view, the definition of comorbidity refers to a situation in which "a distinct clinical entity develops during a disease" (e.g. when a patient with diabetes mellitus develops Parkinson's disease). In this case, there are two distinct clinical entities, and a lifetime concept is applied. Instead, from a clinical point of view the definition of comorbidity refers to a situation in which "two or more distinct clinical entities coexist". In this case, the prevalence of comorbidity depends on the definition of the disorders in question (i.e. the classification system and its diagnostic rules). In the field of mental health, in which specific biomarkers are thus far lacking, it is questionable whether psychiatric illnesses are in fact "distinct" clinical entities, or simply the result of the diagnostic criteria currently being applied to their symptoms. Indeed, reliance to the letter on the Diagnostic and Statistical Manual of Mental Disorders (DSM) classification system being used today, the DSM-5, may encourage the application of several psychiatric diagnoses in the same patient.

Problems related to the definition of comorbidity may have important clinical consequences that affect treatment. For example, the features of depression are common in patients with eating disorders, but may be evidence of either a coexistent clinical depression ("true comorbidity") or the direct consequence of eating disorders ("spurious comorbidity"). In the first case, clinical depression should be treated directly, while in the second case, treating the eating disorder should lead to remission in the depressive features.

Furthermore, uncritical management of comorbidities may have the paradoxical effect of defocusing the treatment from the key factors maintaining the eating disorder psychopathology, and subjecting the patient to treatments that are in fact useless and potentially harmful. Specifically, the most frequent therapeutic error that we have observed in our clinical practice is treating the physical and psychosocial consequences of malnutrition using a variety of drugs, without obtaining any clinical benefit. For example, oestrogen and progestins are prescribed to treat secondary amenorrhoea, anxiolytics, and/or antidepressants, neuroleptics, and mood stabilizers to treat anxiety, irritability, mood deflection, and insomnia—symptoms that are in most cases the consequence of malnutrition and/or the eating disorder psychopathology. Similar therapeutic misjudgements are often made with the adoption of psychological treatments that address the psychosocial consequences of the disorder, but not the specific psychopathology of the eating disorder directly.

The above issues prompted us to write this book to share with clinicians the strategies and procedures we have found useful in and assessing and treating "complex" eating disorder cases. We rely on enhanced cognitive behavioural therapy (CBT-E), an evidence-based treatment recommended for all eating disorder categories in both adults and adolescents, but our strategic and pragmatic approach to the management of the medical and psychiatric comorbidities that often coexist with eating disorders can be used by clinicians who adhere to different theoretical models.

That being said, we strongly suggest that multidisciplinary teams managing complex patients with eating disorders adhere to a coherent theoretical and therapeutic model. To this end, the book describes how we have addressed this challenge, developing an approach called "multistep CBT-E". This is a treatment, based on the evidence-based CBT-E, designed to be delivered at three levels of care (outpatient, day-hospital, and inpatient) by a "non-eclectic" multidisciplinary team in which all members received extensive training on CBT-E and are aware of the entire clinical picture of patients. In the non-eclectic multidisciplinary team, the physician's interventions to treat coexisting mental and general medical disorders (e.g. clinical depression, obesity, diabetes) or complications associated with low weight and/or purging behaviours are integrated consistently with CBT-E and coordinated with the other team members, following the pragmatic guidelines described in this book.

The book is divided into two main parts. Part One describes the eating disorder psychopathology, the limitations of the current classification system, the physical and psychosocial consequences of these disorders, and how to assess their nature and severity—essential knowledge for understanding whether a patient has a true or spurious comorbidity. This is followed by an overview of CBT-E and how to implement it at different levels of care.

Part Two describes the general strategies used to address comorbidity in patients with eating disorders, and the specific strategies and procedures for managing the most common mental disorders (i.e. clinical depression, anxiety disorders, obsessive-compulsive disorder, post-traumatic stress disorder, substance use disorder, and personality disorders) and general medical conditions (i.e. obesity, type 1 diabetes, celiac disease, inflammatory bowel diseases, food allergies, and intolerance) coexisting with eating disorders. A clinical case vignette is provided for each disorder to illustrate the practical application of the strategies used to manage these complex cases.

Finally, the appendices include two validated self-report questionnaires: The Eating Problem Checklist (EPCL) questionnaire, designed to assess the psychopathology of eating disorders; and the Starvation Symptom Inventory (SSI), designed to measure malnutrition symptoms in underweight patients.

We hope that this book will prove a useful guide, not only for all clinicians who treat patients with eating disorders (e.g. psychiatrists, internists, endocrinologists, psychologists, dietitians, nutritionists, nurses, educators, physical therapists), but also for the many (e.g. gynaecologists, endocrinologists, gastroenterologists, haematologists, allergists, psychiatrists, psychotherapists, and psychologists) who, while not working in specialized centres, are involved in the management of medical and psychiatric comorbidities in patients with eating disorders.

Garda, Italy   Riccardo Dalle Grave, MD
Verona, Italy   Massimiliano Sartirana, PsyD
Garda, Italy   Simona Calugi, PhD

Acknowledgements

First and foremost, we would like to thank our esteemed mentor Professor Christopher G. Fairburn, whose ideas inspired us to write this book. Heartfelt thanks also go to all of our colleagues at the Department of Eating and Weight Disorders at Villa Garda Hospital for their valuable suggestions. Additional thanks are also due to Anna Forster for her editing services and professionalism.

Contents

Abbreviations

AN	Anorexia nervosa
BED	Binge-eating disorder
BMD	Bone mineral density
BMI	Body mass index
BN	Bulimia nervosa
CBT	Cognitive behaviour therapy
CBT-E	Enhanced cognitive behaviour therapy
DSM-5	Diagnostic and Statistical Manual of Mental Disorders
ECG	Electrocardiogram
EDE	Eating Disorder Examination
EPCL	Eating Problem Checklist
HbA1c	Glycated haemoglobin
HRQOL	Health-related quality of life
ICD-11	International Classification of Diseases, 11th Revision
IGF-1	Insulin-like growth factor 1
IPT	Interpersonal psychotherapy
MMPI	Minnesota Multiphasic Personality Inventory
NICE	National Institute for Health and Care Excellence
OEDs	Other eating disorders
SSI	Starvation Symptom Inventory
SSRI	Selective serotonin reuptake inhibitor
PTSD	Post-traumatic stress disorder

Part I
Eating-Disorder Psychopathology, Comorbidity, and Cognitive Behaviour Therapy

Chapter 1
Eating Disorders: An Overview

Eating disorders are among the most common and serious health problems afflicting adolescents and young women in Western countries. They are less frequent in men. If not treated quickly and well, they interrupt the normal process of psychological and physical development, and cause considerable physical and psychosocial morbidity [1]. They may also lead to death in some cases [2]. Anorexia nervosa, in particular, has the highest mortality rate of any mental disorder, with a standardized mortality ratio of 5.9 over 12.8 years[1] [3], peaking in the first 10 years of follow-up [4].

1.1 Eating Problems and Eating Disorders

Most people who follow a diet or have binge-eating episodes do not have an eating disorder. The latter develops when the diet is so extreme and rigid, and binge-eating episodes so frequent, as to cause physical and psychological impairment and compromise the quality of life. In other words, alterations in eating behaviour must be of clinical severity for an eating disorder to be diagnosed.

In adults and adolescents, there are three main eating disorders: (i) anorexia nervosa, (ii) bulimia nervosa, and (iii) binge-eating disorder. However, community and clinical studies have shown that a large number of individuals with an eating disorder of clinical severity do not fall into these three categories. Such people have an

---

[1] The standardized mortality ratio is the ratio of observed deaths in the study group to expected deaths in the general population. The SMR may be quoted as either a ratio or a percentage. If the SMR is quoted as a ratio and is equal to 1.0, this means the number of observed deaths equals that of expected cases. If the SMR is greater than 1.0, there is a higher number of deaths than expected.

eating disorder that in this book we have grouped into the broad category "other eating disorders".[2]

1.2   Anorexia Nervosa

According to the fifth edition of the Diagnostic and Statistical Manual of Mental Disorders (DSM-5), a person must meet the following three diagnostic criteria if they are to be diagnosed with anorexia nervosa [5]:

1. Restriction of energy intake relative to requirements, leading to a significant low body weight in the context of age, sex, developmental trajectory and physical health. Significantly low body weight is defined as a weight below that is less than minimally normal or, for children and adolescents, less than that minimally expected.[3]
2. Intense fear of gaining weight or becoming fat, or persistent behaviour that interferes with weight gain, even though at significantly low weight.
3. Disturbance in the way in which one's body weight or shape is experienced, undue influence of body weight or shape on self-evaluation, or persistent lack of recognition of the seriousness of the current low body weight.

The presence of amenorrhoea, a criterion required by the previous DSM versions, is no longer necessary for the diagnosis of anorexia nervosa. This exclusion was justified by the observation that amenorrhoea is not predicted by psychopathological variables, only by body weight and excessive exercising, and that individuals who meet all the other diagnostic criteria of anorexia nervosa but do not have amenorrhoea respond in a similar way to the same treatment [6]. In addition, this criterion cannot be applied to women of pre-menarchal or post-menopausal age, those taking oral contraceptives, or, of course, males.

Indeed, although anorexia nervosa mainly affects female adolescents and young adults, about one in eight cases occurs in males [7]. It occurs more commonly among white populations than in non-Hispanic black and Hispanic populations [8],

---

[2] The Diagnostic and Statistical Manual of Mental Disorders (DSM-5) combines feeding and eating disorders in a single diagnostic category. Feeding disorders mainly, but not exclusively, affect children and adolescents, and include the following diagnostic categories: pica, rumination disorder and avoidant/restrictive food intake disorder. Feeding disorders are not discussed in this book since these states present quite differently from the main eating disorders (i.e., there is an absence of the core overvaluation of shape, weight and their control, and no binge-eating episodes or compensatory behaviors). In addition to anorexia nervosa, bulimia nervosa and binge-eating disorder, the eating disorders include a large group of "other specified or unspecified feeding or eating disorders", which in this book we have grouped into a single category, which we term "other eating disorders".

[3] The threshold for defining a significantly low weight is debated and varies. Body Mass Index or BMI thresholds (kg/m^2) of 17.5, 18.0 or 18.5 are typically used. BMI-for-age growth charts are used to assess BMI in youths.

and its global incidence seems to be increasing, particularly in Asia [9] and the Middle East [10]. The most recent large epidemiological study found that lifetime prevalence of the disorder (i.e., the proportion of anorexia nervosa at any point in life) is approximately 0.80% in the United States [8], affecting 1.4% (0.1–3.6%) of women and 0.2% (0–0.3%) of men, according to a recent review of 33 studies [11].

In such individuals, low weight is achieved by adopting an extreme and rigid hypocaloric diet, sometimes associated with excessive exercising. About a third of people with anorexia nervosa have recurrent binge-eating episodes, many of which are subjective,[4] during which their attempt to restrict food intake is disrupted. Binge-eating episodes are often followed by one or more compensatory behaviours, such as self-induced vomiting and laxative and diuretics misuse.

In some cases, anorexia nervosa is short-lived and goes into remission with a brief course of treatment (especially in adolescents) or no treatment at all, but it tends to persist in many cases, and will require prolonged and complex specialized interventions [12]. In about half of anorexia nervosa cases, there is a migration towards bulimia nervosa and other subthreshold eating disorders [13]. At short-term follow-up, the remission rate is about 29%, which increases to 68–84% at 8- to 16-year follow-up [12]. Unfortunately, however, about 10–20% of sufferers do not improve with any treatment available to date, and develop a lifelong condition [14] that is today is called "severe and enduring" anorexia nervosa [15, 16]. In these cases, the disorder impairs health-related quality of life (HRQOL) more or less markedly and persistently, and is associated with increased need for healthcare and associated costs [17]. The crude mortality rate for anorexia nervosa ranges between 0% and 8%, with the most recent studies reporting a cumulative mortality rate of about 2.8% [12].

1.3 Bulimia Nervosa

Bulimia nervosa, originally known in North America as "bulimia", was first described in 1979 [18]. According to the DSM-5, a person suffers from bulimia nervosa if they meet the following diagnostic criteria [5]:

1. Recurrent episodes of binge eating. An episode of binge eating is characterized by both of the following:

    (a) Eating, in a discrete period of time (e.g., within any 2-h period), an amount of food that is definitely larger than most people would eat during a similar period of time and under similar circumstances.
    (b) A sense of lack of control over eating during the episode (e.g., a feeling that one cannot stop eating or control what or how much one is eating).

---

[4]A small or moderate amount of food associated with sense of lack of control over eating during the episode, as opposed to objective binge-eating episodes, in which the amount of food consumed is, in fact, unusually large.

2. Recurrent inappropriate compensatory behaviour in order to prevent weight gain, such as self-induced vomiting; misuse of laxatives, diuretics, or other medications; fasting; or excessive exercise.
3. The binge eating and inappropriate compensatory behaviours both occur, on average, at least once a week for 3 months.
4. Self-evaluation is unduly influenced by body shape and weight.
5. The disturbance does not occur exclusively during episodes of anorexia nervosa.

Bulimia nervosa mainly affects young women, with a female to male ratio of 1–20 [7]. The lifetime prevalence of bulimia nervosa is 0.28 in the United States [8], being 1.9% (0.3–4.6%) in women and 0.6% (0.1–1.3%) in men according to a recent review of 33 studies [11].

In typical cases, the disorder begins between the ages of 18 and 25 with the adoption of strict and extreme dietary rules, motivated by excessive concerns about shape and weight. In about a quarter of diagnosed cases, there has been a period in which the diagnostic criteria for anorexia nervosa have been met [19]. In bulimia nervosa, the diet is periodically interrupted by binge-eating episodes followed by compensatory behaviours such as self-induced vomiting, laxatives and diuretics misuse, fasting or strict dieting, and/or excessive exercising. The combination of dietary restriction, binge-eating episodes and compensatory behaviours rarely produces a persistent calorie deficit, which explains why individuals with bulimia nervosa are typically in the normal-weight or overweight range.

Although it may vary in severity, once it manifests, bulimia nervosa tends to be self-perpetuating. About 20% of cases migrate to binge-eating disorder or other subthreshold eating disorders, while the transition to anorexia nervosa is less frequent [20]. The remission rates for bulimia nervosa are about 27–28% at 1-year follow-up, and increase as the duration of follow-up increases (up to 70% or more by 10-year follow-up) [12]. More than 20% of patients have a persistent course [20], and in this case, the disorder impairs HRQOL more or less markedly and persistently [17]. Reported crude mortality rates have ranged from 0 to 2% across studies, with a cumulative mortality rate of 0.4% [21].

1.4   Binge-Eating Disorder

As the term suggests, binge-eating episodes are the main feature of binge-eating disorder. This is a relatively recently acknowledged disorder, although people with obesity having recurrent binge-eating episodes were described by Albert Stunkard in 1959 [22]. The DSM-5 diagnostic criteria for binge-eating disorder are as follows [5]:

1. Recurrent episodes of binge eating. An episode of binge eating is characterized by both of the following:

(a) Eating, in a discrete period of time (for example, within any 2-h period), an amount of food that is definitely larger than most people would eat in a similar period of time under similar circumstances.

(b) A sense of lack of control over eating during the episode (for example, a feeling that one cannot stop eating or control what or how much one is eating).

2. The binge-eating episodes are associated with three (or more) of the following:

(a) Eating much more rapidly than normal.
(b) Eating until feeling uncomfortably full.
(c) Eating large amounts of food when not feeling physically hungry.
(d) Eating alone because of feeling embarrassed by how much one is eating.
(e) Feeling disgusted with oneself, depressed, or very guilty afterwards.

3. Marked distress regarding binge eating is present.
4. The binge eating occurs, on average, at least once a week for 3 months.
5. The binge eating is not associated with the recurrent use of inappropriate compensatory behaviour as in bulimia nervosa and does not occur exclusively during the course of bulimia nervosa or bulimia nervosa.

In short, individuals with binge-eating disorder have recurrent binge-eating episodes not followed by a systematic use of compensatory behaviours (e.g., self-induced vomiting, misuse of laxatives or diuretics, fasting, excessive exercising).

For a diagnosis of binge-eating disorder, the International Classification of Diseases 11th Revision (ICD-11)'s definition of a binge-eating episode does not require the intake of food to be excessive. According to the ICD-11, the "binge-eating disorder is characterized by frequent, recurrent episodes of binge eating (e.g., once a week or more over a period of several months). A binge-eating episode is a distinct period of time during which the individual experiences a *subjective* loss of control overeating, eating notably more or differently than usual, and feels unable to stop eating or limit the type or amount of food eaten" [23]. This definition of binge-eating episodes seems more clinically useful than the DSM-5 description because it is in line with the experience reported by patients with binge-eating disorder. Indeed, these generally report that loss of control and perception of having eaten in excess rather than how much food is eaten are more decisive in characterizing the experience of distress associated with a binge-eating episode [24].

The lifetime prevalence of binge-eating disorder is 0.85 in the United States [8], and was reported as 2.8% (0.6–5.8%) in women and 1.0% (0.3–2.0%) in men following a review of 33 studies [11]. Unlike other eating disorders, such as anorexia nervosa and bulimia nervosa, where the female to male ratio is 9:1, in binge-eating disorder the ratio is approximately 6:4 [25]. Furthermore, the disorder is present in all ethnic/racial groups with a similar prevalence [8].

Binge-eating disorder can occur at any age, although it typically starts in late adolescence or young adulthood. The average age of onset is about 21 years [26], but there is a broad distribution of the age of disorder onset that ranges from 14 to 30 years. In typical cases, binge-eating disorder begins with binge-eating episodes, often in association with stressful life events. Binge eating often results in weight gain, and for this reason some individuals make several attempts to lose weight, without, however, in most cases, achieving lasting weight loss. This process is the opposite of what happens in bulimia nervosa, where generally the diet precedes the onset of binge-eating episodes. Moreover, in binge-eating disorder, binge-eating episodes occur in the context of excessive and dysregulated eating rather than dietary restraint and restriction, and this behaviour explains the disorder's strong association with obesity. In some cases, however, the onset of the disorder occurs after a period of strict dieting.

Patients generally report a long history of binge-eating episodes, with an increase in their frequency during times of stress, and also long periods free from this behaviour. Results from drug trials and studies examining the short-term natural history of the disorder indicate that it is characterized by high rates of spontaneous remission [27]. In those who do not achieve remission, migration from this disorder to anorexia nervosa or bulimia nervosa is rare. However, binge-eating disorder increases approximately twofold the risk of developing overweight, obesity, and depression [28].

1.5 Other Eating Disorders

Many eating disorders do not meet the diagnostic criteria for anorexia nervosa, bulimia nervosa, or binge-eating disorder. These disorders have attracted numerous definitions (e.g., eating disorders not otherwise specified, unspecified eating disorders, atypical eating disorders, and, more recently, other specified or unspecified feeding or eating disorders). As previously mentioned, for this book we decided to use the broad term "other eating disorders".

In recent years, this category has attracted a lot of attention from clinicians and researchers because it has been seen that it is much more frequent than previously thought, affecting about 20% of people with eating disorders [29] (Fig. 1.1). In common with anorexia nervosa and bulimia nervosa, the majority of people affected are adolescents or young women.

The DSM-5 describes five other specified feeding or eating disorders [5]:

Fig. 1.1 Pie chart illustrating the relative lifetime prevalence of the four diagnostic categories of eating disorders

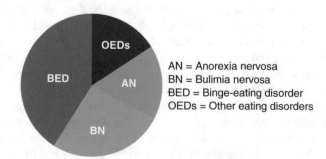

AN = Anorexia nervosa
BN = Bulimia nervosa
BED = Binge-eating disorder
OEDs = Other eating disorders

1. **Atypical anorexia nervosa**: All of the criteria for anorexia nervosa are met, except that despite significant weight loss, the individual's weight is within or above the normal range.
2. **Bulimia nervosa (of low frequency and/or limited duration):** All of the criteria for a diagnosis of bulimia nervosa are met, except that the binge eating and inappropriate compensatory behaviours occur, on average, less than once a week and/or for less than 3 months.
3. **Binge-eating disorder (of low frequency and/or limited duration):** All of the criteria for binge-eating disorder are met, except that the binge eating occurs, on average, less than once a week and/or for less than 3 months.
4. **Purging disorder:** Recurrent purging behaviour to influence weight or shape (e.g., self-induced vomiting, misuse of laxatives, diuretics, or other medications) in the absence of binge eating.
5. **Night eating syndrome:** Recurrent episodes of night eating, as manifested by eating after awakening from sleep or by excessive food consumption after the evening meal. There is awareness and recall of the eating. The night eating is not better explained by external influences such as changes in the individual's sleep–wake cycle or by local social norms. The night eating causes significant distress and/or impairment in functioning. The disordered pattern of eating is not better explained by binge-eating disorder or another mental disorder, including substance use, and is not attributable to another medical disorder or an effect of medication.

Little is known about the course of other eating disorders, which, if defined according to the DSM-5 criteria, seem to have a lifetime prevalence of 1.5% [29]. In most cases, the onset is in adolescence or early adulthood, and about a quarter and a third have a history of anorexia nervosa and bulimia nervosa, respectively, with a similar duration of the disorder. One study has reported that the probability of remission from these eating disorders is about 60% [29].

1.6 The Transdiagnostic Perspective

The DSM-5 classification encourages eating disorders to be considered as distinct entities. This distinction, however, has three main limitations from a treatment perspective (Table 1.1) [30]. The first is that the eating disorders described as separate in the classification in fact share most clinical features; patients in each group have similar eating habits and concerns about body weight and shape. This means that a distinction between the diagnostic categories is sometimes difficult to make, and in any case would be artificial. For example, an adult female with the characteristics of bulimia nervosa and low weight (e.g., BMI = 18.4) would be diagnosed on the basis of her weight, rather than the clinical features of the disorder; if her weight were considered significantly low, she would receive a diagnosis of anorexia nervosa, otherwise the diagnosis would be bulimia nervosa—a state of affairs that would

Table 1.1 The three main limitations of the DSM diagnostic distinctions between eating disorders

1.	Eating disorders share a common eating disorder psychopathology
2.	Many clinical eating disorders do not meet the diagnostic criteria for anorexia nervosa, bulimia nervosa or binge-eating disorder, and instead are grouped under the umbrella category of "other specified or unspecified feeding or eating disorders"
3.	Eating disorders migrate between different diagnostic categories

seem to run counter to clinical wisdom. Another problematic issue is the differential diagnosis between bulimia nervosa and binge-eating disorder; in people who do not vomit or misuse laxatives or diuretics, according to the DSM-5 the distinction between the two disorders is to be determined by the amount of food that they eat between binge-eating episodes; if the amount is small, they will receive a diagnosis of bulimia nervosa; otherwise, it will be classified as binge-eating disorder. In short, there are no clear boundaries between the various diagnostic categories for eating disorders.

The second limitation of the current diagnostic system is that it provides an incomplete picture of the eating disorders that are present in both clinical and community samples. As mentioned, many eating disorders do not meet the diagnostic criteria for anorexia nervosa, bulimia nervosa or binge-eating disorder, and so have been grouped into an umbrella category, namely "other specified or unspecified feeding or eating disorders". This murky situation is further complicated by the third limitation, brought to light by longitudinal studies assessing the course of eating disorders; these have found that they migrate between different eating disorder categories, but only rarely evolve from or into other mental disorders [31]. Indeed, it is not uncommon to observe that a patient who presents at the beginning of the year has one specific eating disorder diagnosis, but 6 months later is eligible for another eating disorder diagnosis, without, however, experiencing any significant change in psychopathology. For example, in our clinical experience we have encountered numerous patients who in adolescence had received a diagnosis of anorexia nervosa, but then after a certain period of time had migrated to bulimia nervosa and/or another eating disorder.

These three limitations of the DSM-5 classification have led to suggestions that eating disorders should, in fact, be considered as different presentations of a single diagnostic entity rather than separate disorders (Fig. 1.2), in a so-called transdiagnostic perspective [30].

For the above reasons, both enhanced cognitive behavioural therapy (CBT-E) and this book are based on this transdiagnostic perspective, which has several clinical and research implications. From a clinical point of view, it calls into question the implication that each DSM-5 diagnostic category will require a specific form of treatment. Indeed, the fact that eating disorders tend to persist and evolve in their clinical characteristics, but do not migrate into other mental disorders, suggests that common transdiagnostic processes play an important role in maintaining the psychopathology of eating disorders [30]. It follows, therefore, that treatments which can address these maintenance processes should be effective with all diagnostic categories of eating

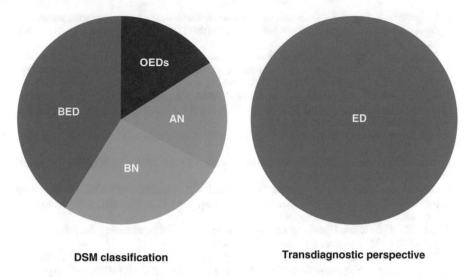

Fig. 1.2 Schematic representation of how eating disorders are classified according to DSM-5 and the transdiagnostic perspective. *AN* Anorexia nervosa, *BN* Bulimia nervosa, *BED* Binge-eating disorder, *OEDs* Other eating disorders, *ED* Eating disorder

disorders. Data collected in recent years on the similar effects of CBT-E as applied to the various diagnostic categories of eating disorders, in both adolescence and adulthood, support the transdiagnostic hypothesis (see Chap. 3). It is hoped that further research into treatment response and natural history of transdiagnostic samples may lead to the development of a less artificial and more clinically useful approach to diagnosis. Meanwhile, in line with the available evidence, in this book patients are considered as sharing a common eating disorder psychopathology.

References

1. Wade TD, Wilksch SM, Lee C. A longitudinal investigation of the impact of disordered eating on young women's quality of life. Health Psychol. 2012;31(3):352–9. https://doi.org/10.1037/a0025956.
2. Crow SJ, Peterson CB, Swanson SA, Raymond NC, Specker S, Eckert ED, et al. Increased mortality in bulimia nervosa and other eating disorders. Am J Psychiatry. 2009;166(12):1342–6. https://doi.org/10.1176/appi.ajp.2009.09020247.
3. Arcelus J, Mitchell AJ, Wales J, Nielsen S. Mortality rates in patients with anorexia nervosa and other eating disorders. A meta-analysis of 36 studies. Arch Gen Psychiatry. 2011;68(7):724–31. https://doi.org/10.1001/archgenpsychiatry.2011.74.
4. Franko DL, Keshaviah A, Eddy KT, Krishna M, Davis MC, Keel PK, et al. A longitudinal investigation of mortality in anorexia nervosa and bulimia nervosa. Am J Psychiatry. 2013;170(8):917–25. https://doi.org/10.1176/appi.ajp.2013.12070868.
5. American Psychiatric Association. Diagnostic and statistical manual of mental disorders, (DSM-5). Arlington: American Psychiatric Publishing; 2013.

6. Dalle Grave R, Calugi S, Marchesini G. Is amenorrhea a clinically useful criterion for the diagnosis of anorexia nervosa? Behav Res Ther. 2008;46(12):1290–4. https://doi.org/10.1016/j.brat.2008.08.007.
7. Steinhausen HC, Jensen CM. Time trends in lifetime incidence rates of first-time diagnosed anorexia nervosa and bulimia nervosa across 16 years in a Danish nationwide psychiatric registry study. Int J Eat Disord. 2015;48(7):845–50. https://doi.org/10.1002/eat.22402.
8. Udo T, Grilo CM. Prevalence and correlates of DSM-5-defined eating disorders in a nationally representative sample of U.S. adults. Biol Psychiatry. 2018;84(5):345–54. https://doi.org/10.1016/j.biopsych.2018.03.014.
9. Pike KM, Dunne PE. The rise of eating disorders in Asia: a review. J Eat Disord. 2015;3:33. https://doi.org/10.1186/s40337-015-0070-2.
10. Mitchell JE, Peterson CB. Anorexia Nervosa. N Engl J Med. 2020;382(14):1343–51. https://doi.org/10.1056/NEJMcp1803175.
11. Galmiche M, Dechelotte P, Lambert G, Tavolacci MP. Prevalence of eating disorders over the 2000–2018 period: a systematic literature review. Am J Clin Nutr. 2019;109(5):1402–13. https://doi.org/10.1093/ajcn/nqy342.
12. Keel PK, Brown TA. Update on course and outcome in eating disorders. Int J Eat Disord. 2010;43(3):195–204. https://doi.org/10.1002/eat.20810.
13. Bulik CM, Sullivan PF, Fear J, Pickering A. Predictors of the development of bulimia nervosa in women with anorexia nervosa. J Nerv Ment Dis. 1997;185(11):704–7. https://doi.org/10.1097/00005053-199711000-00009.
14. Steinhausen HC. The outcome of anorexia nervosa in the 20th century. Am J Psychiatry. 2002;159(8):1284–93. https://doi.org/10.1176/appi.ajp.159.8.1284.
15. Calugi S, El Ghoch M, Dalle Grave R. Intensive enhanced cognitive behavioural therapy for severe and enduring anorexia nervosa: a longitudinal outcome study. Behav Res Ther. 2017;89:41–8. https://doi.org/10.1016/j.brat.2016.11.006.
16. Dalle Grave R. Severe and enduring anorexia nervosa: no easy solutions. Int J Eat Disord. 2020;53:1320–1. https://doi.org/10.1002/eat.23295.
17. Ágh T, Kovács G, Supina D, Pawaskar M, Herman BK, Vokó Z, et al. A systematic review of the health-related quality of life and economic burdens of anorexia nervosa, bulimia nervosa, and binge eating disorder. Eat Weight Disord. 2016;21(3):353–64. https://doi.org/10.1007/s40519-016-0264-x.
18. Russell G. Bulimia nervosa: an ominous variant of anorexia nervosa. Psychol Med. 1979;9(3):429–48.
19. Sullivan PF, Bulik CM, Carter FA, Gendall KA, Joyce PR. The significance of a prior history of anorexia in bulimia nervosa. Int J Eat Disord. 1996;20(3):253–61. https://doi.org/10.1002/(sici)1098-108x(199611)20:3<253::aid-eat4>3.0.co;2-n.
20. Steinhausen HC, Weber S. The outcome of bulimia nervosa: findings from one-quarter century of research. Am J Psychiatry. 2009;166(12):1331–41. https://doi.org/10.1176/appi.ajp.2009.09040582.
21. Keel PK, Mitchell JE. Outcome in bulimia nervosa. Am J Psychiatry. 1997;154(3):313–21. https://doi.org/10.1176/ajp.154.3.313.
22. Stunkard AJ. Eating patterns and obesity. Psychiatry Q. 1959;33(2):284–95. https://doi.org/10.1007/BF01575455.
23. World Health Organization. International classification of diseases for mortality and morbidity statistics (11th Revision); 2018. Available from: https://icd.who.int/browse11/l-m/en.
24. Hay P. Current approach to eating disorders: a clinical update. Intern Med J. 2020;50(1):24–9. https://doi.org/10.1111/imj.14691.
25. Hudson JI, Hiripi E, Pope HG Jr, Kessler RC. The prevalence and correlates of eating disorders in the National Comorbidity Survey Replication. Biol Psychiatry. 2007;61(3):348–58. https://doi.org/10.1016/j.biopsych.2006.03.040.

26. Citrome L. Binge-eating disorder and comorbid conditions: differential diagnosis and implications for treatment. J Clin Psychiatry. 2017;78(Suppl 1):9–13. https://doi.org/10.4088/JCP. sh16003su1c.02.
27. Agras WS, Crow S, Mitchell JE, Halmi KA, Bryson S. A 4-year prospective study of eating disorder NOS compared with full eating disorder syndromes. Int J Eat Disord. 2009;42(6):565–70. https://doi.org/10.1002/eat.20708.
28. Field AE, Sonneville KR, Micali N, Crosby RD, Swanson SA, Laird NM, et al. Prospective association of common eating disorders and adverse outcomes. Pediatrics. 2012;130(2):e289–95. https://doi.org/10.1542/peds.2011-3663.
29. Mustelin L, Lehtokari VL, Keski-Rahkonen A. Other specified and unspecified feeding or eating disorders among women in the community. Int J Eat Disord. 2016;49(11):1010–7. https:// doi.org/10.1002/eat.22586.
30. Fairburn CG, Cooper Z, Shafran R. Cognitive behaviour therapy for eating disorders: a "transdiagnostic" theory and treatment. Behav Res Ther. 2003;41(5):509–28. https://doi. org/10.1016/s0005-7967(02)00088-8.
31. Milos G, Spindler A, Schnyder U, Fairburn CG. Instability of eating disorder diagnoses: prospective study. Br J Psychiatry. 2005;187:573–8. https://doi.org/10.1192/bjp.187.6.573.

Chapter 2
Eating Disorder Psychopathology and Its Consequences

Eating disorders can be considered cognitive disorders because they share a specific core psychopathology that is cognitive in nature. All eating disorder patients overvalue, that is to say ascribe excessive importance to their body shape, weight and/or eating, and devote an unreasonable amount of time and energy to their control [1]. The main expressions of eating disorders, for example strict dieting, significantly low weight, binge-eating episodes, excessive exercising and purging behaviours and the negative physical and psychosocial consequences, all stem either directly or indirectly from this core psychopathology. Each patient may display a variable range of such expressions, and so a clear understanding of the features of eating disorder psychopathology and its consequences is a necessary prerequisite to making an accurate assessment of each patient both at intake and throughout the course of treatment. As part of the assessment process, it is also vital to differentiate between those expressions that arise as part of the eating disorder, and those that are related to other psychiatric disorders and/or general medical diseases.

2.1 Eating Disorder Psychopathology

People who judge themselves predominantly, and in some cases exclusively, on the basis of their body shape and weight, and keeping tight control on the same, are described as overvaluing shape, weight and their control [1, 2]. This contrasts with people without eating disorders, who generally evaluate themselves on the basis of their perceived performance in a variety of life domains, e.g. relationships, work, sport and parenting (Fig. 2.1). The overvaluation of shape and weight and their control should be differentiated from body dissatisfaction as the former is more closely associated with self-esteem than the latter [3], and better differentiates individuals with eating disorders from those without [4].

© The Author(s), under exclusive license to Springer Nature
Switzerland AG 2021
R. Dalle Grave et al., *Complex Cases and Comorbidity in Eating Disorders*,
https://doi.org/10.1007/978-3-030-69341-1_2

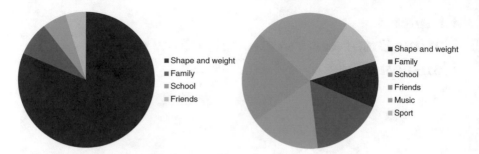

Fig. 2.1 Representative "self-worth" pie chart of a person with an eating disorder (on the left) and without (on the right). Note: the size of the slice corresponds to the relative degree of importance attributed to each domain in self-evaluation

Overvaluation of shape, weight and their control is common to anorexia nervosa and bulimia nervosa, and occurs in more than 50% of patients with binge-eating disorder [5], as well as a large subgroup of patients with other specified eating disorders [6]. Reported by both female and male patients, it is unique to the eating disorders, and is rarely seen in the general population. Hence, the overvaluation of shape, weight and their control can be considered a specific core psychopathology of most eating disorders [1]. This psychopathology is defined as "specific" because it is a common characteristic of the majority of people with an eating disorder but seldom seen in those without. It is the "core" psychopathology because the main clinical features of eating disorders derive directly or indirectly from it.

The most characteristic expressions of overvaluation of shape, weight and their control are *preoccupation with shape and weight*, *body checking* and *body avoidance*. Other specific expressions are *feeling fat*, the *pursuit of thinness* and the *fear of gaining weight*, which are not mitigated by weight loss.

The core psychopathology also explains the extreme weight control behaviours adopted by people with eating disorders; these may include *strict dieting*, *excessive exercising*, *self-induced vomiting* and *laxative and diuretics misuse*. These behaviours may result in a persistent negative energy balance, producing a condition of *low weight*, which, in turn, can lead to the onset of *starvation syndrome*, which is characterized by specific physical and psychosocial symptoms that exacerbate the afflicted person's deteriorating health, and will be described in detail in Sect. 2.2.

The only eating disorder feature that is not apparently a direct expression of the overvaluation of shape, weight and their control is *binge-eating*. However, in many cases binge-eating episodes are the consequence of the strict and extreme dietary rules adopted by people with eating disorders being broken, regardless of whether they produce a significant calorie deficit or not.

In a subgroup of people with eating disorders, the core psychopathology consists of the *overvaluation of eating control* per se. Such individuals do not report the fear of gaining weight or extreme concerns about shape and weight, but are solely preoccupied with eating control. Sometimes this psychopathology coexists with the overvaluation of shape and weight, but not always. Like overvaluation of shape and

Table 2.1 The main expressions of eating disorder psychopathology

- Overvaluation of shape, weight and their control
- Overvaluation of eating control
- Preoccupation with shape, weight and eating
- Fear of weight gain
- Pursuit of thinness
- Strict dieting
- Binge-eating episodes
- Self-induced vomiting
- Misuse of laxatives
- Misuse of diuretics
- Excessive exercising
- Food checking
- Body checking
- Body avoidance
- Feeling fat
- Low weight and starvation symptoms

weight, overvaluation of eating control per se is expressed via the adoption of strict and extreme dietary rules, and frequent and unusual food checking (e.g. repeatedly weighing food and checking the calorie content of food to be eaten). This condition is particularly common in young adolescents, who in some cases may receive a DSM-5 diagnosis of avoidant/restrictive food intake disorder [7]. Table 2.1 shows the main expressions of the specific psychopathology common to eating disorders.

2.1.1 Eating Problem Check List: A Questionnaire for Assessing Eating Disorder Psychopathology

The Eating Problem Check List (EPCL) is a 16-item tool designed to assess eating disorder behaviours and psychopathology over the previous 7 days [8]. It is quick and easy to complete, and can be readily integrated into routine clinical practice. Specifically, the EPCL can be used in the assessment phase to assess the eating disorder psychopathology, and during treatment to assess how this changes from week to week. It is also suitable for use in research evaluating the effects of treatment. Indeed, through weekly assessment of the two subscale scores—Body Image and Eating Concerns—the EPCL can help to evaluate the changes in the core psychopathology of eating disorders. Furthermore, by weekly monitoring of each single-item score, the clinician can promptly focus treatment on specific expressions of a patient's individual eating disorder psychopathology.

The EPCL, what it is, how it is designed to be used, its validation status and score assignment are presented in Appendix A.

2.2   The Effects of Calorie Restriction and Low Weight

The Minnesota Starvation Experiment is the most important study to evaluate the effects of undereating and weight loss in normal-weight people, and it is particularly relevant for understanding eating disorders because many of the physical, but especially psychological and social, symptoms observed in its healthy participants are similar to those experienced by people with eating disorders who are underweight [9]. The study was conducted by Ancel Keys and collaborators at the University of Minnesota between 19 November 1944 and 20 December 1945 [10]. It was designed to assess the physiological and psychological effects of severe and prolonged dietary restriction and the effectiveness of nutritional rehabilitation strategies. The principal aim of the investigators was to collect information to improve the management of famine victims in Europe and Asia during and after World War II by using the data derived from a laboratory simulation of severe famine.

More than 100 men volunteered for the study as an alternative to military service. The participants were all young adult white males (age range 22–33 years). The 36 men selected had both the best physical and psychological health and the greatest commitment to the experimental objectives. Of the 36 volunteers, 25 were members of the Historic Peace Churches (Mennonites, Church of the Brethren and Quakers).

The study was divided into three phases: (i) a control period of 12 weeks; (ii) 24 weeks of semi-starvation and (iii) 12 weeks of rehabilitation. During the control period the mean daily energy intake of the participants was 3492 calories; during the period of semi-starvation this was decreased to a mean of 1570 calories, and during the rehabilitation period it was raised back to normal levels. In the semi-starvation period, participants were fed foods most likely consumed in European famine areas, and lost approximately 25% of their body weight. A subgroup was followed up for almost 9 months after the nutritional rehabilitation phase had begun. Most of the results were reported for only 32 men as four of the participants in the experiment dropped out either during or at the end of the caloric restriction phase. Although individual responses to weight loss varied greatly, all men experienced dramatic physical, psychological and social changes, which are summarized in the following sections.

2.2.1   Behavioural Effects

Many of the behaviours reported in the Minnesota Starvation Experiment will be familiar to clinicians who have observed underweight patients with an eating disorder. For example, towards the end of the semi-starvation period, participants spent 2 h eating a meal that would have only taken a few minutes to consume in the control period. They also spent hours planning how to divide up their prescribed amount of daily food. Nineteen of the 36 began reading cookbooks and collecting recipes. Participants tried to keep their stomachs full by drinking large amounts of fluid (water and soups). Many also increased their consumption of coffee and tea, with some drinking more than 15 cups a day. They asked that the food be served hot, mixed food in strange ways, and increased their application of salt and spices. Their consumption of chewing gum—for some participants even as much as 40 packets a day—smoking, and onychophagy (nail biting) increased markedly. Many of these changes persisted even after the 12 weeks of weight restoration.

During the semi-starvation period, all participants reported an increase in hunger; some were able to tolerate it, while for others it became unbearable. Several of the participants failed to adhere to the prescribed diet and experienced binge-eating episodes, which they then criticized themselves for. During the weight-restoration phase, when they were offered a large amount of food, many participants seemed to lose "normal" control, eating either more or less than necessary. Increased hunger was even reported after a large meal at 12 weeks of rehabilitation. In most cases, normalization of eating habits occurred only after about 5 months of rehabilitation, but in some participants the excess food consumption continued beyond that. The factor discriminating between those whose eating habits normalized and those who continued to eat large amounts of food was not identified.

In general, participants responded to calorie restriction with a reduction in their physical activity. They became tired, weak, inattentive and apathetic, and complained of a lack of energy. The movements of the volunteers became considerably slower. However, some participants occasionally practised spontaneous exercise. Some tried to lose more weight by trying to expend more energy so that they would be provided a more abundant bread ration, or to avoid a further reduction in rations. This attitude is similar to the practice of some people with eating disorders who, if they believe they have exercised more strenuously, feel that they can afford to eat more. The difference is that for those who suffer from eating disorders, calorie restriction is self-imposed.

2.2.2   Psychological Effects

Many Minnesota Starvation Experiment participants, although initially psychologically healthy, showed marked cognitive and emotional changes during and after the semi-starvation period. In particular, they reported decreased concentration capacity, insight and critical judgement, even though no objective changes in intellectual ability were observed. It is likely therefore that their impaired concentration capacity was due to the presence of recurrent thoughts about food and eating reported by most of the participants.

In addition, some participants suffered transient or prolonged bouts of depression, while others displayed periods of euphoria followed by depression. Although all volunteers had demonstrated high stress tolerance prior to the study, many exhibited frequent signs of irritability and outbursts of anger. In many participants the anxiety was very evident, and apathy became common. In some, emotional disorders became so severe as to be labelled as "semi-starvation neurosis". The observed and reported emotional changes were confirmed by the Minnesota Multiphasic Personality Inventory (MMPI), which showed a significant increase in depression, hysteria, and hypochondria—the so-called neurotic triad commonly observed in neurotic individuals. Moreover, two participants developed psychotic symptoms, and one self-mutilated three fingers of his hand to modulate his mood. In general, the emotional changes did not disappear immediately after rehabilitation, but persisted for many weeks.

The study shows that the emotional response to calorie restriction varies considerably from individual to individual, and that personality does not predict the emotional response to semi-starvation. Since some emotional difficulties did not resolve immediately during the rehabilitation phase, it can be assumed that these alterations were related not only to caloric restriction but also to low body weight levels. This suggests that many of the psychological disorders observed in underweight people with eating disorders may, in fact, be the simple result of undereating and low weight, rather than an integral part of the disorder.

2.2.3 Social Effects

Semi-starvation also had a dramatic effect on social functioning. Participants become inward-looking and self-focused, which led to social withdrawal. In addition, they reported a marked decrease in sexual interest, masturbation and erotic fantasies. These changes are similar to those observed in underweight patients with eating disorder, who tend to become socially isolated, lose their desire for sex and avoid contact with their partner.

2.2.4 Physical Effects

After 6 months of semi-starvation, participants reported various physical changes, including abdominal pain, difficult and long digestion, sleep disturbances, vertigo, headache, strength reduction, hypersensitivity to light and noises, oedema, cold intolerance, sight and hearing alterations and paraesthesia ("pins and needles"). Participants showed a marked reduction in their basal metabolism (almost a 40% decrease), as well as decreased pulse rate and respiratory frequency. During the weight-restoration phase, after having lost 25% or more of their initial body weight, their basal metabolic rate increased proportionally with their increased energy intake, and they regained their baseline body weight; in fact, on average weight levels increased by 10%, but then gradually returned to baseline. This result shows that the body cannot be simply "reprogrammed" to a lower weight after a period of weight loss, and that the volunteers' experimental dietary restriction failed to overcome the strong propensity of their bodies to return to their baseline body weight [11]. Table 2.2 provides a summary of the effects of semi-fasting reported by Minnesota Starvation Experiment participants.

Table 2.2 Summary of the effects reported by Minnesota starvation experiment participants

Behavioural effects
- Food rituals (eating very slowly, cutting food into small pieces, mixing food bizarrely, ingesting boiling food)
- Reading cookbooks and collecting recipes
- Increased consumption of coffee, tea, spices, chewing gum and water
- Onychophagy
- Increased cigarette smoking
- Binge-eating episodes
- Increased exercise to avoid further reductions in calorie content of the diet
- Self-harm

Psychological effects
- Impaired concentration
- Poor critical judgement
- Preoccupation with food
- Depression
- Mood swings
- Irritability
- Anger
- Anxiety
- Apathy
- Rigidity
- Indecision
- Procrastination

Social effects
- Social withdrawal
- Reduced sexual desire

Physical changes
- Sleep disorders
- Dizziness
- Weakness
- Abdominal pain
- Gastrointestinal disorders
- Headache
- Hypersensitivity to noise and light
- Oedema
- Hypothermia
- Reducing heart rate and breathing
- Paraesthesia
- Increased hunger
- Early sense of fullness

2.2.5   Comments from Minnesota Starvation Experiment Participants

In 2003–2004, 18 of the 36 participants still alive were interviewed by researchers from The Johns Hopkins University School of Medicine [12]. Participants were in their 80s when interviewed, and each spoke passionately when discussing why they had chosen to be a conscientious objector and participate in the experiment. Although the study data had been reported in scientific detail in *The Biology of Human Starvation* book, this interview gave participants an opportunity to provide vivid personal accounts of their daily lives during the experiment [12]. In particular, they described that, after their initial enthusiasm, during the semi-starvation period they experienced great changes in personality. They became more irritable and impatient towards others, and began to feel more socially withdrawn. They also reported suffering from the physical effects of calorie restriction, describing a lack of energy, dizziness, extreme fatigue, cold intolerance, muscle soreness, hair loss, reduced coordination, ringing in their ears and poor concentration. Food became an obsession, and many lost interest in sex. Despite these difficulties, they reported that they remained strongly determined to continue the experiment, and gave different reasons for their dedication (including religious reasons, discipline and will-power) [12].

Interestingly, some participants considered the rehabilitation period to be the most difficult part of the experiment. Some reported that the symptoms of dizziness, apathy and lethargy were the first to dissipate, while the feeling of fatigue, loss of sexual desire and weakness took much longer to improve. Many overate after the experiment ended, and put on excess weight. In general, they reported not being able to return to their usual activities even after 3 months of rehabilitation, and the average time for them to achieve a full recovery ranged from 2 months to 2 years. That being said, none of the participants believed that the experiment had provoked a deleterious effect in the long term [12].

2.2.6   Implications for Psychopathology Assessment

As we have seen, the Minnesota Starvation Experiment findings highlight how many symptoms thought to be specific to anorexia nervosa are in fact secondary to undereating and low weight [13]. These symptoms are not all food and weight related, but potentially extend to all areas of social and psychological functioning [11]. Since many symptoms postulated as integral to eating disorders are actually secondary to calorie restriction and being underweight, it follows that normalizing body weight is essential for normal psychological function and personality to be restored [11].

That being said, in individuals with eating disorders the effects of being underweight are different to those observed in subjects without these disorders. In people who are required by circumstances to undereat for prolonged periods of time, starvation symptoms have the adaptive function of prolonging life by reducing basal metabolism and focusing the attention of the individuals primarily on the search for food. When food becomes available, starving people eat without being concerned about losing control of their shape and weight. This, however, does not happen in people with eating disorders [14]. In fact, two studies have shown that in such individuals the effects of caloric restriction and being underweight seem to reinforce, or "maintain", eating disorder psychopathology [15, 16]. For example, when they interact with eating disorder psychopathology, some starvation symptoms are interpreted by patients as a threat to their control over eating (e.g. hunger potentially prompting them to eat more than they had planned) or as their failure to control their food intake (e.g. the early sense of fullness being seen as a sign that they have over-eaten). Other starvation symptoms, such as social withdrawal, reinforce the condition by inducing them to isolate from external "normal" experiences that could serve to reduce their overvaluation of shape, weight and eating control by introducing/reinforcing other self-evaluation domains (Fig. 2.2). Finally, some patients may interpret some starvation symptoms (e.g. hunger, dizziness, weakness and feeling cold) in a positive light, seeing them as signs of their success in controlling eating and weight.

2.2.7   Starvation Symptom Inventory: A Questionnaire for Assessing Starvation Symptoms

As we have seen, many of the symptoms ascribed to eating disorders are, in fact, the consequences of their undereating. The Starvation Symptom Inventory (SSI) is designed to assess the psychosocial and physical symptoms of starvation, as discussed in the preceding section, in patients suffering from eating disorders. It is a questionnaire consisting of 15 items pertaining to the last 28 days [17], and, like the EPCL, can be used in both the assessment phase and during treatment to monitor change due to weight regain and nutritional rehabilitation. Likewise, it is also suitable for use in research into the effects of treatments for eating disorders. The SSI, what it is, how it should be used, its validation status and score assignment are presented in Appendix B.

2.3   The Psychosocial Consequences of Eating Disorder Psychopathology

The psychopathology of eating disorders (i.e. overvaluation of shape, weight and their control, strict dieting, excessive exercising, binge-eating episodes and/or purging behaviours), regardless of whether or not weight is low, impairs the

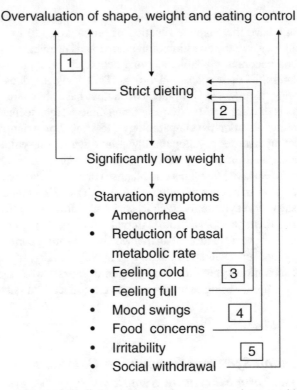

Fig. 2.2 How some low weight, dieting, and starvation symptoms interact with eating-disorder psychopathology

1 = Significantly low weight and strict dieting are not seen as a problem, but rather as achievements (in presence of the overvaluation of shape, weight, and their control)

2 = Reduction in basal metabolic rate leads to a slowdown in weight loss, which suggests an inability to control weight and leads to tighter calorie restriction

3 = Food concerns cause them to make their diet even more rigid

3 = Feeling full is interpreted as having eaten too much and prompts intensification of dieting

4 = Social withdrawal prevents experiences that can help reduce the importance attributed to shape, weight, and eating control

psychological and interpersonal functioning of affected individuals. Most are irritable, depressed and demoralized, and many are ashamed of their perceived lack of willpower and feel guilty about their behaviour. Self-criticism is common, and some sufferers become so desperate that they attempt suicide. Others engage in self-harm to punish themselves for their uncontrolled behaviour and/or to relieve tension.

The presence of a depressed mood is common and, when not associated with being underweight, is generally the consequence of binge-eating episodes, tending to resolve when the person regains control of their diet. In a subgroup of patients, however, a coexisting clinical depression can develop (see Chap. 5), distinguished by the presence of certain typical characteristics. These include the onset or accentuation of a depressed mood tone in the absence of changes in the eating disorder features, a general loss of interest, thoughts of death, recurrent crying episodes and social isolation [18]. Some people with eating disorders, especially those with recurrent binge-eating episodes, misuse alcohol when experiencing mood changes.

Many people with eating disorders are anxious, both as a character trait, and, especially, when they encounter situations that trigger their concerns about shape, weight and eating control. Typically, they tend to avoid social situations involving eating, such as birthday parties or friends' weddings, and also situations that require some degree of body exposure, such as going to the pool or the beach, as well as changing rooms and revealing their body to a partner.

Two personality traits are prominent in people with eating disorders [1]. The first is *low self-esteem*. Feelings of inadequacy and low self-worth are common and, despite often being part of their general demoralization or depression, tend to improve with remission of their eating disorder psychopathology. In some cases, however, these feelings are expressions of their own personality traits and precede the eating disorder onset.

The other common personality trait seen in individuals with an eating disorder is *perfectionism* [1]. Many people with eating disorders tend to set extremely demanding standards for themselves, and their perfectionism tends to affect all aspects of their lives, being particularly evident in their efforts to control energy intake. Although this trait may have some positive aspects, helping them to excel at school, work or other areas of life they deem important, in most cases, and particularly when their standards are unrealistic and unachievable, it may have negative consequences. If this happens, the repeated experience of failure to meet their very high personal standards can undermine their self-worth, even if their performance is in reality above average or excellent.

In the worst cases, the eating disorder psychopathology negatively affects all aspects of the lives of people with eating disorders. The overvaluation of shape, weight and their control leads to harmful behaviours such as strict dieting, excessive exercising and binge-eating, which inevitably occupy most of the day. As a consequence, relationships with family and friends become fractured. However, most interpersonal problems, along with depression, low self-esteem, anxiety and irritability, improve markedly with the remission of eating disorder psychopathology.

2.4   The Physical Consequences of Eating Disorder Psychopathology

Physical complications are common in patients with eating disorders, and are the result of four main mechanisms, often operating in concert, namely *dietary restriction*, *being underweight*, *excessive exercising* and *purging* (i.e. self-reported vomiting or misuse of laxatives and diuretics) [19, 20]. Luckily, most of the physical consequences are reversed with timely remission of the eating disorder psychopathology. Table 2.3 describes the main physical manifestations observed in eating disorders.

Table 2.3 Main physical consequences of eating disorder psychopathology

Physical signs
• Arrest of breast growth or non-development (if the onset is pre-pubertal)
• Bradycardia (heart rate <60 beats/min), hypotension (systolic <90 mmHg)
• Hypothermia, cold and cyanotic hands and feet
• Dry skin, lanugo on the back, forearms and sides of the face, yellow-orange colouring of palms and toes
• Telogen effluvium (i.e. extensive hair loss, without the appearance of hairless patches)
• Petechiae (i.e. small—1–2 mm—Red or purple spot on the skin)
• Erosion of the inner surfaces of the teeth (in those who induce vomiting)
• Fragile nails
• Oedema (ankles, pretibial and periorbital regions)
• Weakness of the proximal muscles (difficulty in getting up from a squatting position)
Gastrointestinal complications
• Gastroesophageal reflux, oesophagitis, haematemesis (in those who self-induce vomiting)
• Gastroparesis, gastric dilation and rupture (rarely, in those with binge-eating episodes)
• Decrease in colon motility
• Alterations in liver function enzymes
• High levels of amylases (especially in those who self-induce vomiting)
Endocrine and metabolic complications
• Low levels of oestradiol (in females) and testosterone (in males); low or low normal triiodothyronine (T3) and thyroxine (T4) levels with normal, low or slightly increased thyroid stimulating hormone (TSH), but not as high as it would be in hypothyroidism (euthyroid sick syndrome); hypercortisolism with high levels of free urinary cortisol; increased concentration of growth hormone with low levels of insulin-like growth factor (IGF-1)
• Hypoglycaemia, hypercholesterolemia
• Hypokalaemia and low manganese (especially in those who adopt purging behaviours)
• Low phosphate (especially during refeeding), hyponatremia (especially in those with excessive water intake)
• Osteopenia and osteoporosis (with increased risk of fractures)
Haematological complications
• Anaemia, leukopenia, neutropenia, thrombocytopenia
Cardiovascular complications
• ECG anomalies (especially in those with electrolyte disorders)—low voltage, long QT interval, U waves
Kidney complications
• Kidney stones
Reproductive complications
• Amenorrhea, delayed puberty
• Infertility
• Insufficient weight gain during pregnancy and low birth weight
Neurological complications
• Enlargement of the cerebral ventricles and cerebrospinal spaces (pseudoatrophy)
• Peripheral neuropathy

References

1. Fairburn CG, Cooper Z, Shafran R. Cognitive behaviour therapy for eating disorders: a "transdiagnostic" theory and treatment. Behav Res Ther. 2003;41(5):509–28. https://doi.org/10.1016/s0005-7967(02)00088-8.
2. Fairburn CG. Cognitive behavior therapy and eating disorders. New York: Guilford Press; 2008.
3. Masheb RM, Grilo CM. The nature of body image disturbance in patients with binge eating disorder. Int J Eat Disord. 2003;33(3):333–41. https://doi.org/10.1002/eat.10139.
4. Goldfein JA, Walsh BT, Midlarsky E. Influence of shape and weight on self-evaluation in bulimia nervosa. Int J Eat Disord. 2000;27(4):435–45.
5. Grilo CM, White MA, Gueorguieva R, Wilson GT, Masheb RM. Predictive significance of the overvaluation of shape/weight in obese patients with binge eating disorder: findings from a randomized controlled trial with 12-month follow-up. Psychol Med. 2013;43(6):1335–44. https://doi.org/10.1017/s0033291712002097.
6. Dalle Grave R, Calugi S. Transdiagnostic cognitive behavioural theory and treatment of body image disturbance in eating disorders: a guide to assessment, treatment, and prevention. In: Cuzzolaro M, Fassino S, editors. Body image, eating, and weight. Cham: Springer; 2018.
7. American Psychiatric Association. Diagnostic and statistical manual of mental disorders, (DSM-5). Arlington: American Psychiatric Publishing; 2013.
8. Dalle Grave R, Sartirana M, Milanese C, El Ghoch M, Brocco C, Pellicone C, et al. Validity and reliability of the eating problem checklist. Eat Disord. 2019;27(4):384–99. https://doi.org/10.1080/10640266.2018.1528084.
9. Dalle Grave R, Pasqualoni E, Marchesini G. Symptoms of starvation in eating disorder patients. In: Preedy VR, editor. Handbook of behavior, food and nutrition. New York: Springer Science+Business Media; 2011. p. 2259–69.
10. Keys A, Brozek J, Henschel A, Mickelsen O, Taylor H. The biology of human starvation. Minneapolis: University of Minnesota Press; 1950.
11. Garner DM. Psychoeducational principles in treatment. In: Garner DM, Garfinkel P, editors. Handbook of treatment for eating disorders. New York: Guilford Press; 1977. p. 145–77.
12. Kalm LM, Semba RD. They starved so that others be better fed: remembering Ancel Keys and the Minnesota experiment. J Nutr. 2005;135(6):1347–52. https://doi.org/10.1093/jn/135.6.1347.
13. Garner DM, Dalle Grave R. Terapia cognitivo comportamentale dei disturbi dell'alimentazione. Verona: Positive Press; 1999.
14. Dalle Grave R, Calugi S. Cognitive behavior therapy for adolescents with eating disorders. New York: Guilford Press; 2020.
15. Dalle Grave R, Di Pauli D, Sartirana M, Calugi S, Shafran R. The interpretation of symptoms of starvation/severe dietary restraint in eating disorder patients. Eat Weight Disord. 2007;12(3):108–13. https://doi.org/10.1007/BF03327637.
16. Shafran R, Fairburn CG, Nelson L, Robinson PH. The interpretation of symptoms of severe dietary restraint. Behav Res Ther. 2003;41(8):887–94.
17. Calugi S, Miniati M, Milanese C, Sartirana M, El Ghoch M, Dalle Grave R. The starvation symptom inventory: development and psychometric properties. Nutrients. 2017;9(9):967. https://doi.org/10.3390/nu9090967.
18. Fairburn CG, Cooper Z, Waller D. Complex cases and comorbidity. In: Fairburn CG, editor. Cognitive behavior therapy and eating disorders. New York: Guilford Press; 2008.
19. Katzman DK. Medical complications in adolescents with anorexia nervosa: A review of the literature. Int J Eat Disord. 2005;37(Suppl):S52–9; discussion S87–9. https://doi.org/10.1002/eat.20118.
20. Westmoreland P, Krantz MJ, Mehler PS. Medical complications of anorexia nervosa and bulimia. Am J Med. 2016;129(1):30–7. https://doi.org/10.1016/j.amjmed.2015.06.031.

Chapter 3
Enhanced Cognitive Behaviour Therapy for Eating Disorders

Enhanced cognitive behaviour therapy (CBT-E) is a personalized transdiagnostic psychological treatment for all eating disorder categories (i.e. anorexia nervosa, bulimia nervosa, binge-eating disorder and other eating disorders). CBT-E was first designed to treat adults in an outpatient setting [1], but versions were later developed for adolescents [2] and intensive levels of care, such as day hospital and inpatient units [3, 4]. The effectiveness of CBT-E is supported by the results of numerous controlled and cohort studies, and the treatment has been recommended by the latest National Institute for Health and Care Excellence (NICE) guidelines as suitable for all adult and adolescents with eating disorders [5].

3.1 Transdiagnostic Cognitive Behavioural Theory

As mentioned above, CBT-E is based on the transdiagnostic cognitive behavioural conceptualization of eating disorders. Cognitive behavioural theory was initially applied to eating disorders by Fairburn in the early 1980s to elucidate and treat bulimia nervosa; the treatment he proposed mainly focused on the processes that maintained the disorder [6, 7]. Subsequently, the theory was extended to explain the transdiagnostic maintenance processes observed to operate in all eating disorders, and the treatment was improved to address four additional external maintenance processes that, in some patients, interact with the eating disorder psychopathology and thereby constitute great obstacles to change [1]. The transdiagnostic theory accounts for the range of processes that maintain any eating disorder diagnostic category, irrespective of its presentation.

R. Dalle Grave et al., *Complex Cases and Comorbidity in Eating Disorders*, https://doi.org/10.1007/978-3-030-69341-1_3

3.2   Core Maintenance Processes

The theory maintains that a distinctive self-evaluation scheme, i.e. the overvaluation of shape and/or weight and/or eating and their control, is of central importance in maintaining eating disorders, irrespective of their classification [1]. Indeed, as we have seen in Chap. 2, most of the other clinical features of eating disorders derive directly or indirectly from this specific core psychopathology. For example, extreme weight-control behaviours (strict dieting, excessive exercising, self-inducing vomiting, misusing laxatives or diuretics), as well as body checking or avoidance, feeling fat, preoccupation with shape, weight, and eating and marginalization of other areas of life, are explained if a person believes that control of shape, weight and eating is of paramount importance in their self-evaluation.

The various clinical expressions of eating disorders derived from the overvaluation of shape, weight, eating and their control maintain the core psychopathology in a state of continuous activation, with the result that the eating disorder mindset becomes locked in place [1, 8]. As mentioned in Chap. 2, the only behaviour characteristic of eating disorders not directly determined by the core psychopathology is binge eating. Present in a subgroup of people suffering from eating disorders, these episodes do, however, tend to stem indirectly from the overvaluation of shape, weight, eating and their control because they are largely triggered and maintained by failed attempts to adhere to self-imposed extreme and rigid dietary rules and/or severe undereating. People with eating disorders tend to react in an extremely negative way (often taking an "all or nothing" stance) to the almost inevitable breaking of their own rules, and in this mindset even a small transgression tends to be interpreted as evidence of poor self-control and personal weakness [9]. The reaction to this perceived lack of self-control is often temporary abandonment of efforts to restrict the diet, resulting in a binge-eating episode. This, in turn, maintains the core eating disorder psychopathology by intensifying concerns about being unable to control shape, weight and eating, and encourages further dietary restriction, thus increasing the risk of further binge-eating episodes.

Three other processes help to maintain binge-eating episodes [9]: (i) life difficulties and associated emotional changes may act as disinhibitors, facilitating breaking of extreme and rigid dietary rules because it is difficult to maintain dietary restraint under such circumstances; (ii) since the binge-eating episode temporarily improves mood and distracts from problems, it may become a dysfunctional means of coping with such difficulties; and (iii) self-induced vomiting or other compensatory behaviours tend to maintain binge-eating episodes because the false belief that such behaviours are effective in preventing calorie absorption removes a major deterrent to binge eating (i.e. the fear of gaining weight).

For those people who meet the DSM-5 diagnostic criteria for anorexia nervosa, binge-eating episodes are predominantly subjective or absent. In these cases, the undereating and low weight predominate, leading to the onset of starvation symptoms [10], which in turn help to maintain the eating disorder through various processes (see Chap. 2). For example, delayed gastric emptying resulting from malnutrition produces an early sense of fullness, even after eating modest amounts of food. Social withdrawal secondary to starvation, on the other hand, intensifies the use of shape and weight as a means of self-evaluation. What is more, the preoccupation with eating is intensified by caloric restriction, and in turn prompts the individual to adopt even more extreme and rigid dietary rules [11, 12].

Figure 3.1 shows the composite transdiagnostic "formulation" describing the main specific maintenance processes operating in eating disorders. The transdiagnostic formulation, or conceptualization, can be adapted to all diagnostic categories of these disorders, or rather to individual manifestations of the eating disorder psychopathology, with minimal changes; it provides a useful guide, to be shared with patients, on the processes that will be addressed by treatment. For example, the formulation of a person with bulimia nervosa does not contain the box "low weight and starvation symptoms" but may include all other characteristics described in the transdiagnostic array of possible eating disorder symptoms. In contrast, the formulation of a patient with anorexia nervosa restricting type will always include the box "low weight and starvation symptoms", but the "binge-eating" and "self-induced vomiting and/or misuse of laxatives" boxes will be omitted. Finally, a patient with anorexia nervosa of the binge-eating/purging type requires the inclusion of the largest number of maintenance processes, while those of binge-eating disorder have the smallest number.

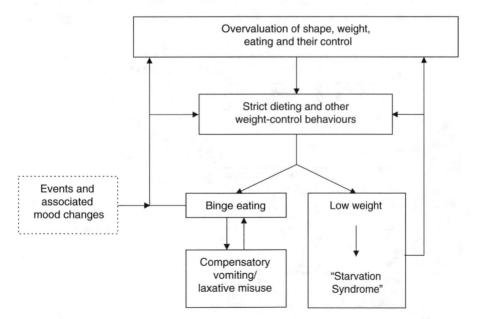

Fig. 3.1 The core processes involved in the maintenance of eating disorders according to transdiagnostic cognitive behavioral theory
Adapted from Fairburn CG, Cooper Z, Shafran R. Cognitive behaviour therapy for eating disorders: A "transdiagnostic" theory and treatment. Behav Res Ther. 2003;41(5):509–28. doi:https://doi.org/10.1016/s0005-7967(02)00088-8. Reprinted with the permission of Elsevier

3.3   Additional Maintenance Processes

In addition to the core eating disorder maintenance processes, transdiagnostic cognitive behavioural theory proposes that one or more of the following additional or "external" mechanisms may be operating in a subgroup of patients (Fig. 3.2) [1]: (i) clinical perfectionism, (ii) core low self-esteem, (iii) marked interpersonal difficulties and (iv) mood intolerance. Additional maintenance mechanisms, if present and marked, interact with the core processes, perpetuating the eating disorder and hindering its treatment.

Clinical perfectionism is an example of dysfunctional self-evaluation similar to the core psychopathology of eating disorders (see Chap. 5, Sect. 5.1). In essence, it refers to overvaluation of achievement and achieving demanding personal standards, despite the adverse consequences [2, 13]. When clinical perfectionism coexists with an eating disorder, there is an interaction between the two psychopathologies because the individual's self-evaluation system focuses on the commitment to trying to achieve "perfect" control of shape, weight and eating, as well as in pursuing demanding standards in other domains of life (e.g. performance in work or sport). Clinical perfectionism also intensifies some aspects of the psychopathology of eating disorder (e.g. dieting and/or excessive exercising), making it more difficult to treat [2, 13].

Core low self-esteem, on the other hand, is characterized by a pervasive negative valuation of self-worth which is not affected by either the events or changes in the

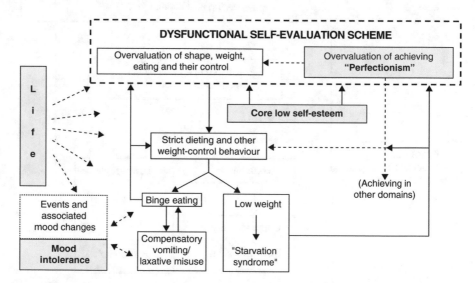

Fig. 3.2 Composite transdiagnostic formulation of eating disorders with additional maintenance processes. "Life" is shorthand for interpersonal life
Adapted from Fairburn CG, Cooper Z, Shafran R. Cognitive behaviour therapy for eating disorders: a "transdiagnostic" theory and treatment. Behav Res Ther. 2003;41(5):509–28. Reprinted with the permission of Elsevier

state of the eating disorder [1]. This extreme form of negative self-evaluation maintains the eating disorder psychopathology through two main processes (see Chap. 5, Sect. 5.2) [2]: (i) it creates a sense of helplessness and a lack of confidence in the ability to change, negatively influencing treatment adherence; and (ii) it encourages the individual to pursue success in some areas that are judged important to improve their self-esteem (e.g. control of shape, weight and eating) with particular determination, thereby making it even more difficult to enact change in these areas.

Marked interpersonal difficulties maintain eating disorder psychopathology through various processes (see Chap. 5, Sect. 5.3). Examples include the following [1]:

- Family tensions may intensify dietary restriction, especially in younger patients. A process that reflects the intensification of their need to have a sense of control is shifted to control over eating [14].
- Some interpersonal environments (e.g. school and family) intensify concerns about control over shape, weight and eating.
- Adverse interpersonal events and associated emotional changes can affect eating control and promote binge-eating episodes.
- Persistent interpersonal difficulties may undermine self-esteem and prompt patients to struggle even harder to achieve certain "positive" goals such as success in controlling shape, weight and eating.

Finally, mood intolerance is defined as the inability to tolerate intense moods, or excessive sensitivity to mood states (see Chap. 5, Sect. 5.4) [1]. People with this psychopathology, when experiencing a change in their emotions, tend to manage it using "dysfunctional mood-modulation behaviours", such as excessive alcohol intake, substance misuse or self-harming behaviours (e.g. cutting or burning the skin, etc.). Moreover, when the psychopathology of eating disorder coexists, they may also use binge-eating, self-induced vomiting and excessive exercising, as means to modulate mood.

3.4 CBT-E: An Overview

CBT-E is a time-limited, personalized psychological treatment for eating disorder psychopathology, rather than a particular eating disorder diagnosis. It is derived from the cognitive behavioural transdiagnostic theory described above, which focuses on the processes maintaining the psychopathology—the real targets of treatment. It was originally designed for adult outpatients of both sexes with a BMI of between 15.0 and 39.9 [1, 15], but was subsequently also adapted for adolescents [2, 16–18] and intensive settings of care [3], such as day-hospital and inpatient units, where patients with severe eating disorders and/or BMI <15 are generally treated. The management of patients with eating disorder psychopathology and a BMI equal to or greater than 40 is described in another publication [19].

3.4.1 Treatment Goals

CBT-E has four major goals [2]:

1. To engage patients in the treatment and involve them actively in the process of change;
2. To remove the eating disorder psychopathology, i.e. dietary restraint and restriction (and low weight if present), extreme weight-control behaviours, and preoccupation with shape, weight and eating;
3. To correct the mechanisms maintaining the eating disorder psychopathology;
4. To ensure lasting change.

3.4.2 General Strategies

CBT-E is designed to be a comprehensive treatment, and should not be combined with other forms of psychotherapy. It is a specific form of cognitive behaviour therapy (CBT), and, like many empirically supported forms of CBT, is a time-limited treatment that addresses the processes that maintain the patient's psychopathology.

Unlike other treatments applied in eating disorders [20], which postulate that the illness stems from the patient (externalization), and therefore promote therapists or parents "taking control" of the patient, CBT-E treats the problem as *belonging* to the individual. As such, it treats the illness as part of the individual, and encourages the patient, rather than therapists or parents, to take control.

Indeed, all CBT-E procedures are designed to make patients feel in control, actively involving them in the decision of whether or not to start treatment, and the choice of problems to be targeted and the procedures used to address them. The therapist informs the patients that overcoming the eating disorder will be difficult, but worth it, and treatment should therefore be given priority in their lives. The therapist also ensures that the patients understand what is going on at any point in the treatment, and encourages them to become active participants in the process of achieving change. In short, CBT-E is a collaborative means of overcoming the eating disorder psychopathology (collaborative empiricism). Hence CBT-E never adopts "prescriptive" or "coercive" procedures; in other words, patients are never asked to do things that they do not agree to, as this may increase their resistance to change [18].

A key strategy of CBT-E is to collaboratively create with the patients a personalized formulation (or set of hypotheses) of the main processes of maintaining their eating disorder psychopathology, which will become the targets of treatment (Fig. 3.1). The personalized formulation is the basis for a tailored treatment addressing a patient's individual evolving psychopathology. The formulation helps the patient to visualize the mechanisms at play, and can be modified during the treatment to address any emerging processes. The patients are educated about the processes reported on the formulation, and are actively involved in the decision to address each of them. If they do not conclude that they have a problem to address, the treatment cannot start or must be postponed for a time, but this is a rare occurrence.

Once patients are engaged in the process of change, their eating disorder psychopathology is addressed via a flexible set of sequential cognitive and behavioural strategies and procedures, integrated with ongoing education. Two main principles guide CBT-E: (i) simpler procedures are preferred over more complex ones, and (ii) it is better to do a few things well rather than many things badly (the principle of parsimony). As in other forms of CBT, self-monitoring and success in completing strategically planned homework tasks between sessions are of paramount importance. Since these can create anxiety, the therapist needs to be not only empathetic but also aware of when and how to keep the patient firmly on track.

Although CBT-E relies upon a variety of generic cognitive behavioural strategies and procedures (e.g. addressing cognitive biases such as dichotomous thinking and selective attention in the usual way), it differs from generic CBT in several aspects. For example, conventional thought recording is not used throughout, though patients are asked to record their thoughts and feelings about particular topics at certain points (e.g. when addressing feeling fat and/or body checking) in the last column of their CBT-E self-monitoring records. Furthermore, CBT-E does not often use formal cognitive restructuring or make reference to other certain widely used CBT concepts, namely automatic thoughts, assumptions, core beliefs and schemas [15]. In patients with eating disorder psychopathology, we do not find these methods or concepts necessary to produce the required changes. CBT-E also makes limited use of formal behavioural experiments as these tend to be hard to interpret in patients with eating disorders. In any case, the outcomes of greatest relevance to the core eating disorder psychopathology (i.e. changes in the overvaluation of shape, weight, eating and their control) do not lend themselves to short-term experimentation, and so different strategies are preferred.

As part of CBT-E, it is considered essential that patients learn to de-centre from their eating disorder [15]. For this purpose, in the first phase of the treatment patients are prompted to make gradual behavioural changes and analyse the effects and implications of these on their way of thinking. This approach usually produces a gradual reduction in their preoccupation with shape, weight, eating and their control. In the later stages of the treatment, when the main maintenance processes have been disrupted and the patients report experiencing periods free from shape, weight and eating concerns, the treatment focuses on helping them to recognize the early warning signs of eating disorder mindset reactivation, and to de-centre from it quickly, thereby averting relapse.

3.4.3   Forms of CBT-E

CBT-E can be administered in two forms: (i) the "focused" form, which addresses only the core maintenance processes of the eating disorder psychopathology; and (ii) the "broad" form, which uses specific modules to address one or more of the additional maintenance processes (i.e. clinical perfectionism, core low self-esteem, marked interpersonal difficulties and/or mood intolerance). The focused form is indicated for most patients, while the broad form is introduced only when the external maintenance processes are pronounced, seem to be acting to maintain the eating disorder psychopathology, and interfere with the treatment. The decision to use the broad form is taken in a review session held after 4 weeks in not-underweight patients, or in one of the review sessions later on in underweight patients.

3.4.4   Adaptations for Clinical Groups and Settings

CBT-E has been adapted for adults and adolescents, and can be delivered in the following four settings, or levels of care: (i) outpatient, (ii) intensive outpatient, (iii) inpatient and (iv) post-inpatient outpatient.

3.4.4.1   Outpatient CBT-E

The outpatient version is recommended for most adult patients with eating disorders. As evaluated in trials, CBT-E is a time-limited treatment, with 20 weeks generally given to non-underweight patients and 40 weeks to underweight patients [15]. Although imposing time limitations on CBT-E might be seen to affect its personalized nature, there are considerable advantages to a fixed timeframe that outweigh such disadvantages. In particular, a set time-limit helps both the patient and the therapist to focus on working hard to help the patient change, and facilitates the development of the "therapeutic momentum". It also increases the likelihood of the treatment having a formal ending, thereby overcoming the uncertainty of more open-ended treatments. Finally, it ensures that future-oriented topics that are fundamental to a patient's long-term remission will be addressed in the final sessions.

In some cases, the treatment needs to be shortened, for example in patients with binge-eating disorder if the binge eating rapidly ceases and there is little other psychopathology to address. More often, however, a case can be made for extending treatment. Examples include when the treatment has been disrupted (e.g. by clinical depression or an interpersonal crisis), or when patients who benefit but are still significantly impaired experience a setback not long after the treatment has ended. Under these circumstances, the treatment should be continued for some additional months, with a detailed review of the progress being held every 4 weeks to ensure that continuance is justified.

CBT-E for *non-underweight patients* is divided into four "Stages" designed to address the eating disorder psychopathology of such patients (Fig. 3.3). In Stage One, the focus is on gaining a mutual understanding of the person's eating problem and helping him or her to modify and stabilize their pattern of eating. There is also an emphasis on personalized education and addressing an individual's concerns about weight. It is best if these initial sessions are twice a week. In Stage Two, the

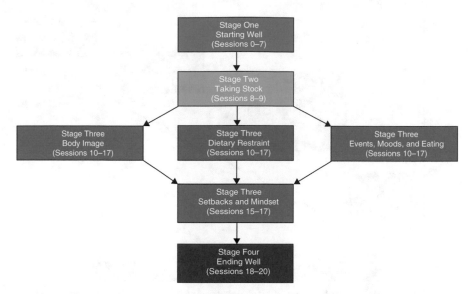

Fig. 3.3 CBT-E Map for non-underweight patients, i.e., with a BMI of 18.5–39.9 (20 sessions over 20 weeks)

Reproduced with permission from the Online Training Programme in CBT-E, CREDO Oxford, 2017

progress is systematically reviewed, and plans are made for the main body of treatment (Stage Three). Stage Three consists of a run of weekly sessions focused on the processes that are maintaining the person's eating problem. Usually, this involves addressing concerns about shape, weight and eating, enhancing their ability to deal with day-to-day events and moods, and addressing extreme dietary restraint. Towards the end of Stage Three and throughout Stage Four the emphasis shifts to preparing for the future, with a focus on dealing with setbacks and maintaining the changes that have been achieved. Generally, a review session is held 20 weeks after treatment has ended. This provides an opportunity for reviewing progress and addressing any problems that remain or have emerged.

With *underweight patients*, treatment needs to be longer, often involving around 40 sessions over 40 weeks. In this version of CBT, the process of achieving weight gain is articulated over three "Steps" (Fig. 3.4): Step One focuses on deciding to address weight regain, Step Two on regaining a healthy weight, and Step Three on maintaining weight and preventing relapse. In our clinical experience, underweight patients appreciate this approach, finding the three steps easy to understand and implement. In particular, as they tend not to see being underweight as a problem, they appreciate that in Step One the goal is not weight regain but instead to collaboratively evaluate the implications of change. Indeed, in CBT-E the objective is that patients themselves decide to regain weight rather than having this decision imposed upon them, and, during the final Step, that they become accomplished at maintaining their healthier weight.

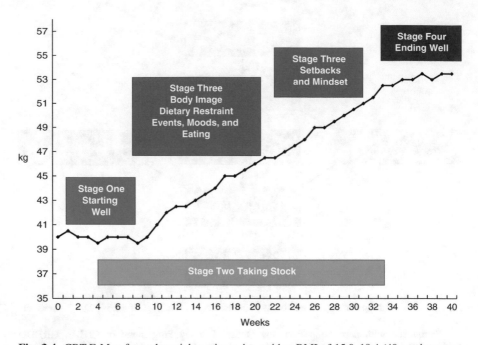

Fig. 3.4 CBT-E Map for underweight patients, i.e., with a BMI of 15.0–18.4 (40 sessions over 40 weeks)
Reproduced with permission from the Online Training Programme in CBT-E, CREDO Oxford, 2017

CBT-E has also been adapted for *adolescents*, taking into account two distinctive characteristics of this population, namely potential implications for long-term physical health, and parental involvement [2]. Indeed, some medical complications associated with eating disorders (e.g. osteopenia and osteoporosis) are particularly severe in this age range, and periodic medical assessments and a lower threshold for hospital admission are therefore integral parts of CBT-E for adolescents. Like the adult version, the programme lasts 20 weeks in not-underweight patients, but in underweight patients the "standard" 40 weeks may be shortened to about 30 weeks, as adolescents tend to restore a normal body weight faster than adults [21]. Parental involvement in the treatment is required in the great majority of cases [2]. Parents are asked to attend an interview lasting approximately 90 min alone during the first week of the treatment, and patient and parents are subsequently seen together in sessions 4–6 (in patients who are not underweight) or sessions 8–10 (in underweight patients). These joint sessions are held 15–20-min immediately after patient session. Table 3.1 describes the core elements of the adolescent's version of CBT-E for underweight patients.

Table 3.1 The core elements of the focused CBT-E version for underweight adolescent patients

Step One—Starting well and deciding to change

The aims are to engage the patient in treatment and change, including addressing weight regain.

The appointments are twice weekly for 4 weeks and involve the following:

- Jointly creating a formulation of the processes maintaining the eating disorder;
- Establishing real-time self-monitoring of eating and other relevant thoughts and behaviours;
- Educating about: body weight regulation and fluctuations, the adverse effects of dieting, and, if applicable, the ineffectiveness and physical complications of self-induced vomiting and laxative misuse as a means of weight control;
- Introducing and establishing weekly in-session weighing, and becoming proficient in interpreting and coping with weight fluctuations;
- Introducing and adhering to a pattern of regular eating, with planned meals and snacks;
- Thinking about addressing weight regain;
- Involving parents to facilitate treatment.

Step two—Addressing the change

The aim is to address weight regain and the key mechanisms that are maintaining the patient's eating disorder.

The appointments are twice a week until the rate of weight regain stabilizes, at which time they are held once a week. This step involves the following CBT-E modules:

- Underweight and Undereating: creating a daily positive energy balance of about 500 kcal to achieve a mean weekly weight regain of about 0.5 kg;
- Overvaluation of Shape and Weight: providing education on overvaluation and its consequences; nurturing previously marginalized domains of self-evaluation; reducing unhelpful body checking and avoidance; re-labelling unhelpful thoughts or feelings such as "feeling fat"; exploring the origins of the overvaluation and learning to identify and control the eating disorder mindset;
- Dietary Restraint: changing inflexible dietary rules into flexible guidelines and introducing previously avoided foods;
- Events and Mood-related Changes in Eating: developing proactive problem-solving skills to tackle such triggering events, and developing skills to accept and modulate intense moods;
- Setbacks and mindsets: Providing education about setbacks and mindsets; identifying eating-disorder mindset reactivation triggers; spotting setbacks early on; displacing the mindset; exploring the origins of the overvaluation.

Review sessions

These are held 1 week after Step One and then every 4 weeks, for the purposes of:

- Collaboratively reviewing progress and treatment compliance;
- Identifying barriers to change, both general (e.g. school pressures) and features of the eating disorder itself (e.g. difficulties in weight regain, presence of dietary restraint);
- Adjusting the initial formulation in light of progress and/or emerging issues;
- Deciding to continue with the focused form of CBT-E rather than the broad form.[a]

Step 3—Ending well

The aims are to ensure that progress made during treatment is maintained, and that the risk of relapse is minimized. There are three appointments, 2 weeks apart, covering the following:

(continued)

Table 3.1 (continued)

• Addressing concerns about ending treatment;
• Devising a short-term plan for continuing to implement changes made during treatment (e.g. reducing body checking, introducing further avoided foods, eating more flexibly, maintaining involvement in new activities) until the post-treatment review session;
• Phasing out treatment procedures, in particular self-monitoring and in-session weighing;
• Education about realistic expectations and identifying and addressing setbacks;
• Devising a long-term plan for maintaining body weight, and averting and coping with setbacks.
Post-treatment review session
• Reviewing the long-term maintenance plan around 4, 12, and 20 weeks after treatment has been finished.

[a]The broad form of CBT-E includes four additional modules (i.e. clinical perfectionism, low self-esteem, interpersonal difficulties, or mood intolerance), one of which may be added to the focused modules in Step Two. This form of treatment is indicated if clinical perfectionism, low self-esteem, interpersonal difficulties, or mood intolerance are marked, and appear to be maintaining the disorder and obstructing change (see Sect. 3.4.4.5 and Chap. 5).

3.4.4.2 Intensive Outpatient CBT-E

This treatment level is designed for patients who may need greater input than outpatient CBT-E can provide, but whose condition is not sufficiently severe as to warrant hospitalization. Intensive outpatient programmes implement all the procedures and strategies of outpatient CBT-E, and also include several features developed specifically for this approach [3, 22]. The intensive treatment lasts for a maximum of 12 weeks, but may be shorter if patients successfully make progress in the areas in which they were struggling with outpatient CBT-E (e.g. lack of weight regain, failure to reduce episodes of binge-eating or eat regular meals). Patients usually spend weekdays in the unit, but the treatment can be flexibly adapted to both the clinical needs of the patient and the logistical limitations of the clinical service that delivers the treatment. However, in our view the optimal programme should include the following procedures on weekdays: (i) supervised daily meals, (ii) individual CBT-E twice weekly, (iii) sessions with a CBT-E trained dietitian to plan and review weekend meals and (iv) regular reviews with a CBT-E-trained physician. Towards the end of intensive treatment, patients who have responded well are gradually encouraged to eat meals outside the unit, thereby allowing the treatment to evolve into conventional outpatient CBT-E.

3.4.4.3 Inpatient CBT-E

Inpatient CBT-E is indicated for patients who have not responded well to the less intensive versions, or as a first-line option for those who require close medical supervision. It is designed to ensure a unified, rather than eclectic, approach to a patient's treatment. The inpatient programme maintains all the main strategies and procedures of CBT-E, which are delivered in both individual sessions and a group format, but has three main features that distinguish it from the outpatient version [3, 22]. Specifically, rather than a single therapist, the treatment is delivered by a multidisciplinary team comprising physicians, psychologists, dietitians and nurses, all fully trained in CBT-E. Secondly, assistance with eating is provided in the first weeks of treatment to help patients get over their difficulties in real time. Thirdly, opportunities are provided for adolescent patients to continue their studies as an integral part of their stay in hospital.

Inpatient CBT-E also includes additional elements designed to reduce the high rate of relapse that typically follows discharge from hospital. For instance, the inpatient unit is open, and patients are free to come and go. This ensures that they continue to be exposed to the types of environmental stimuli that tend to provoke their eating disorder psychopathology, but have full access to staff support. Indeed, during the weeks immediately preceding discharge, a concerted effort is made to identify any likely environmental setback triggers and address them during the individual CBT-E sessions. Furthermore, towards the end of treatment, the significant others of patients are helped to create a positive, stress-free home environment in readiness for their return.

3.4.4.4 Post-Inpatient Outpatient CBT-E

Post-inpatient outpatient CBT-E was designed to reduce the relapse rate that is associated with discharge from hospital, preparing patients for their transition from intensive care and returning to their home environment. Post-inpatient outpatient therapy provides 20 sessions across 20 weeks, with a higher frequency of appointments in the first month after hospitalization (two sessions per week). The main objectives of post-inpatient outpatient CBT-E are helping patients to maintain the changes achieved during their hospitalization, to deal with the difficulties that occur once they return home, and to prevent relapse by identifying and addressing the residual maintenance and control mechanisms at play.

3.4.4.5 Broad CBT-E

Focused CBT-E is the appropriate version of the treatment for most patients. The decision to use the broad version is taken in Stage Two, when the patient and therapist have reviewed the progress achieved in Stage One, or one of the review sessions performed every 4 weeks in underweight patients. At this stage of treatment, the therapist is generally aware of the main obstacles to treatment that will need to be addressed. In line with clinical experience and data available from research, broad CBT-E is recommended when one or more of the following additional maintenance mechanisms are pronounced, maintain the eating disorder and hinder change (all three conditions must be met):

- Clinical perfectionism
- Low nuclear self-esteem
- Marked interpersonal difficulties
- Mood intolerance

After deciding to include a module (we recommend not including more than one module so as not to make the treatment too complex), Stage Three addresses both the eating disorder psychopathology and the additional maintenance mechanism, allocating roughly half the session to each. The content of the four modules is described in Chap. 5, while the treatment guides can be consulted for a more detailed description [2, 23].

3.4.5 CBT-E Clinical Services

The Department of Eating and Weight Disorders at Villa Garda Hospital has developed an innovative treatment model based entirely on CBT-E; it is designed to treat adults and adolescents of all diagnostic categories of eating disorders at three levels of care (outpatient, intensive outpatient and inpatient). The treatment, the effectiveness of which has been validated by our team in numerous studies published in peer-reviewed scientific journals [16, 21, 24–34], is designed to overcome the main problems facing traditional clinical services for eating disorders, such as the use of non-evidence-based psychological treatments, the excessive emphasis on hospitalization, and offering patients completely different types of treatment, in terms of both theory and content, in the transition from the different levels of care (e.g. from outpatient to inpatient and vice versa). Indeed, such "eclectic" approaches disrupt the continuity of care and, understandably, disorientate patients as to which strategies and procedures to use to address their eating disorder psychopathology.

The original and innovative feature of Villa Garda's approach, also called "multistep CBT-E" (Fig. 3.5), is the application of coherent strategies and procedures—based on a single theory and evidence-based CBT-E—at every level of care. The only difference between these levels is the intensiveness of treatment, which is less intensive in the outpatient setting and more intensive in the inpatient setting. Patients who do not respond to outpatient treatment and those whose physical condition

Fig. 3.5 The four levels of multistep CBT-E for eating disorders

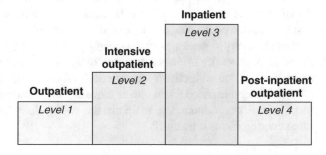

does not warrant hospitalization are offered either intensive outpatient CBT-E or inpatient CBT-E (if hospitalization is indicated). In this way, patients can transition from outpatient to inpatient, and then to post-inpatient outpatient care, without changes to the nature of their treatment.

A clinical service such as the one developed at Villa Garda has two main advantages over traditional clinical services. First, patients are treated with a single, well-delivered, evidence-based treatment, rather than the evidence-free eclectic approach common elsewhere. Second, it minimizes the problems associated with transitions from outpatient to intensive treatment as it avoids subjecting patients to the confusing and counterproductive changes in therapeutic approach that commonly accompany such transitions. However, a different form of treatment must be offered to any patients who do not respond to CBT-E.

In recent years, the promising results of this treatment have attracted the attention of many specialists and, with the supervision of the Villa Garda group, services similar to that offered at Villa Garda Hospital have also been implemented in several countries around the world.

Each level of care is based on the same theory and uses similar strategies and procedures (more intensive in intensive outpatient and inpatient CBT-E).

3.4.6 The Current Status of CBT-E

CBT-E has been tested in all diagnostic categories of eating disorders, in studies in England, Australia, Denmark, Germany, Italy and the USA. The results and the different studies showed some variability in the response rate which may be due to differences in patient samples and the quality of treatment provided. It is striking that the best results were obtained from studies where there was the supervision of the Oxford group and an accurate assessment of how the treatment was administered. These studies were carried out in England (Oxford and Leicester), Denmark (Copenhagen), USA (Minneapolis, St. Paul), and Italy (Verona-Garda).

If one focus on studies in which CBT-E was delivered well, the evidence suggests that with patients who are not significantly underweight, about 80% complete treatment and among them, about two-third achieve a full remission that appears well maintained over time. A large number of the remaining patients improve but do not achieve remission. The rate of remission is similar with underweight patients, but treatment is completed by about 65% of cases.

In general, the research findings can be summarised as follows:

- CBT-E is suitable for treating all diagnostic categories of eating disorders in adult [29, 32, 35] and adolescent subjects [16, 28, 36]. This is not true of any other treatment.
- CBT-E in bulimia nervosa was superior to all the psychological treatments it was compared with, including psychoanalytic psychotherapy and interpersonal therapy [35, 37, 38].

- CBT-E has shown promising results for the outpatient treatment of adult patients with anorexia nervosa [29, 39], and also with those with severe and extreme anorexia nervosa [33].
- CBT-E has shown promising results for the treatment of adolescent patients and from anorexia nervosa and appears to be a potential alternative to family-based treatment [16, 31, 34, 40].
- CBT-E can be used with promising results, particularly in adolescents, in inpatient settings [26, 27, 30, 41]. The inpatients CBT-E appears to be effective also for patients with severe and enduring anorexia nervosa [24, 42].
- To achieve optimal effects, therapists need to be properly trained in CBT-E.

3.4.7   Training in CBT-E

Learning and implementing CBT-E is not difficult for experienced professionals, but the treatment must be taken seriously and should be considered as a "work in progress" that requires continuous practice. Our firm advice is to study the CBT-E manuals for adults [15] and adolescents [2], to carry out online training in CBT-E, which is available free of charge, and to receive supervision by a member of the CBT-E Training Group. Full CBT-E training is also provided in some countries (e.g. the advanced training course in the treatment and prevention of eating disorders and obesity held in Italy has trained more than 450 therapists in CBT-E). For therapists who are not native-English speakers, introductory CBT-E workshops in their languages would be beneficial if no full CBT-E training course is available. Information on online training, clinical CBT-E workshops, and supervision can be obtained from the CBT-E website (www.cbte.co).

References

1. Fairburn CG, Cooper Z, Shafran R. Cognitive behaviour therapy for eating disorders: a "transdiagnostic" theory and treatment. Behav Res Ther. 2003;41(5):509–28. https://doi.org/10.1016/s0005-7967(02)00088-8.
2. Dalle Grave R, Calugi S. Cognitive behavior therapy for adolescents with eating disorders. New York: Guilford Press; 2020.
3. Dalle Grave R. Intensive cognitive behavior therapy for eating disorders. Nova: Hauppauge, NY; 2012.
4. Dalle Grave R. Multistep cognitive behavioral therapy for eating disorders: theory, practice, and clinical cases. New York: Jason Aronson; 2013.
5. National Institute for Health and Care and Clinical Excellence: eating disorders: recognition and treatment I Guidance and guidelines I NICE; 2017. https://www.nice.org.uk/guidance/ng69.
6. Fairburn C. A cognitive behavioural approach to the treatment of bulimia. Psychol Med. 1981;11(4):707–11. https://doi.org/10.1017/s0033291700041209.

7. Fairburn CG, Cooper Z, Cooper PJ. The clinical features and maintenance of bulimia nervosa. In: Brownell KD, Foreyt JP, editors. Physiology, psychology and treatment of the eating disorders. New York: Basic Books; 1986.
8. Teasdale JD. Metacognition, mindfulness and the modification of mood disorders. Clin Psychol Psychother. 1999;6(2):146–55. https://doi.org/10.1002/(sici)1099-0879(199905)6:2<146::Aid-cpp195>3.0.Co;2-e.
9. Cooper Z, Dalle Grave R. Eating disorders: Transdiagnostic theory and treatment. In: Hofmann SG, Asmundson GJG, editors. The science of cognitive behavioral therapy. San Diego: Academic Press; 2017. p. 337–57.
10. Dalle Grave R, Pasqualoni E, Marchesini G. Symptoms of starvation in eating disorder patients. In: Preedy VR, editor. Handbook of behavior, food and nutrition. New York: Springer Science+Business Media; 2011. p. 2259–69.
11. Dalle Grave R, Di Pauli D, Sartirana M, Calugi S, Shafran R. The interpretation of symptoms of starvation/severe dietary restraint in eating disorder patients. Eat Weight Disord. 2007;12(3):108–13. https://doi.org/10.1007/BF03327637.
12. Shafran R, Fairburn CG, Nelson L, Robinson PH. The interpretation of symptoms of severe dietary restraint. Behav Res Ther. 2003;41(8):887–94. https://doi.org/10.1016/s0005-7967(02)00101-8.
13. Shafran R, Cooper Z, Fairburn CG. Clinical perfectionism: a cognitive-behavioural analysis. Behav Res Ther. 2002;40(7):773–91. https://doi.org/10.1016/s0005-7967(01)00059-6.
14. Fairburn CG, Shafran R, Cooper Z. A cognitive behavioural theory of anorexia nervosa. Behav Res Ther. 1999;37(1):1–13. https://doi.org/10.1016/s0005-7967(98)00102-8.
15. Fairburn CG. Cognitive behavior therapy and eating disorders. New York: Guilford Press; 2008.
16. Dalle Grave R, Calugi S, Doll HA, Fairburn CG. Enhanced cognitive behaviour therapy for adolescents with anorexia nervosa: an alternative to family therapy? Behav Res Ther. 2013;51(1):R9–R12. https://doi.org/10.1016/j.brat.2012.09.008.
17. Dalle Grave R, Cooper Z. Enhanced cognitive behavior treatment adapted for younger patients. In: Wade T, editor. Encyclopedia of feeding and eating disorders. Singapore: Springer Singapore; 2016. p. 1–8.
18. Dalle Grave R. Cognitive-behavioral therapy in adolescent eating disorders. In: Hebebrand J, Herpertz-Dahlmann B, editors. Eating disorders and obesity in children and adolescents. Philadelphia: Elsevier; 2019. p. 111–6.
19. Dalle Grave R, Sartirana M, El Ghoch M, Calugi S. Adapting CBT-OB for binge-eating disorder. Treating obesity with personalized cognitive behavioral therapy. Cham: Springer; 2018. p. 195–210.
20. Lock J, Le Grange D. Treatment manual for anorexia nervosa: a family-based approach. 2nd ed. New York: Guilford Press; 2013.
21. Calugi S, Dalle Grave R, Sartirana M, Fairburn CG. Time to restore body weight in adults and adolescents receiving cognitive behaviour therapy for anorexia nervosa. J Eat Disord. 2015;3:21. https://doi.org/10.1186/s40337-015-0057-z.
22. Dalle Grave R, Bohn K, Hawker D, Fairburn CG. Inpatient, day patient and two forms of outpatient CBT-E. In: Fairburn CG, editor. Cognitive behavior therapy and eating disorders. New York: Guilford Press; 2008. p. 231–44.
23. Fairburn CG, Cooper Z, Shafran R, Bohn K, Hawker DM. Clinical perfectionism, core low self-esteem and interpersonal problems. In: Fairburn CG, editor. Cognitive behavior therapy and eating disorders. New York: The Guilford Press; 2008. p. 197–221.
24. Calugi S, El Ghoch M, Dalle Grave R. Intensive enhanced cognitive behavioural therapy for severe and enduring anorexia nervosa: a longitudinal outcome study. Behav Res Ther. 2017;89:41–8. https://doi.org/10.1016/j.brat.2016.11.006.
25. Dalle Grave R, Pasqualoni E, Calugi S. Intensive outpatient cognitive behaviour therapy for eating disorder. Psychol Top. 2008;17(2):313–27. UDC: 616.89-008.441.42-08.

26. Dalle Grave R, Calugi S, Conti M, Doll H, Fairburn CG. Inpatient cognitive behaviour therapy for anorexia nervosa: a randomized controlled trial. Psychother Psychosom. 2013;82(6):390–8. https://doi.org/10.1159/000350058.

27. Dalle Grave R, Calugi S, El Ghoch M, Conti M, Fairburn CG. Inpatient cognitive behavior therapy for adolescents with anorexia nervosa: immediate and longer-term effects. Front Psych. 2014;5:14. https://doi.org/10.3389/fpsyt.2014.00014.

28. Dalle Grave R, Calugi S, Sartirana M, Fairburn CG. Transdiagnostic cognitive behaviour therapy for adolescents with an eating disorder who are not underweight. Behav Res Ther. 2015;73:79–82. https://doi.org/10.1016/j.brat.2015.07.014.

29. Fairburn CG, Cooper Z, Doll HA, O'Connor ME, Palmer RL, Dalle Grave R. Enhanced cognitive behaviour therapy for adults with anorexia nervosa: a UK-Italy study. Behav Res Ther. 2013;51(1):R2–8. https://doi.org/10.1016/j.brat.2012.09.010.

30. Dalle Grave R, Conti M, Calugi S. Effectiveness of intensive cognitive behavioral therapy in adolescents and adults with anorexia nervosa. Int J Eat Disord. 2020;53(9):1428–38. https://doi.org/10.1002/eat.23337.

31. Dalle Grave R, Sartirana M, Calugi S. Enhanced cognitive behavioral therapy for adolescents with anorexia nervosa: outcomes and predictors of change in a real-world setting. Int J Eat Disord. 2019;52(9):1042–6. https://doi.org/10.1002/eat.23122.

32. Fairburn CG, Cooper Z, Doll HA, O'Connor ME, Bohn K, Hawker DM, et al. Transdiagnostic cognitive-behavioral therapy for patients with eating disorders: a two-site trial with 60-week follow-up. Am J Psychiatry. 2009;166(3):311–9. https://doi.org/10.1176/appi.ajp.2008.08040608.

33. Calugi S, Sartirana M, Frostad S, Dalle Grave R. Enhanced cognitive behavior therapy for severe and extreme anorexia nervosa: an outpatient case series. Int J Eat Disord. 2020; https://doi.org/10.1002/eat.23428.

34. Le Grange D, Eckhardt S, Dalle Grave R, Crosby RD, Peterson CB, Keery H, et al. Enhanced cognitive-behavior therapy and family-based treatment for adolescents with an eating disorder: a non-randomized effectiveness trial. Psychol Med. 2020:1–11. https://doi.org/10.1017/s0033291720004407.

35. Fairburn CG, Bailey-Straebler S, Basden S, Doll HA, Jones R, Murphy R, et al. A transdiagnostic comparison of enhanced cognitive behaviour therapy (CBT-E) and interpersonal psychotherapy in the treatment of eating disorders. Behav Res Ther. 2015;70:64–71. https://doi.org/10.1016/j.brat.2015.04.010.

36. Dalle Grave R, Sartirana M, Sermattei S, Calugi S. Treatment of eating disorders in adults versus adolescents: similarities and differences. Clin Ther. 2020; https://doi.org/10.1016/j.clinthera.2020.10.015.

37. Poulsen S, Lunn S, Daniel SI, Folke S, Mathiesen BB, Katznelson H, et al. A randomized controlled trial of psychoanalytic psychotherapy or cognitive-behavioral therapy for bulimia nervosa. Am J Psychiatry. 2014;171(1):109–16. https://doi.org/10.1176/appi.ajp.2013.12121511.

38. de Jong M, Schoorl M, Hoek HW. Enhanced cognitive behavioural therapy for patients with eating disorders: a systematic review. Curr Opin Psychiatry. 2018;31(6):436–44. https://doi.org/10.1097/YCO.0000000000000452.

39. Byrne S, Wade T, Hay P, Touyz S, Fairburn CG, Treasure J, et al. A randomised controlled trial of three psychological treatments for anorexia nervosa. Psychol Med. 2017;47(16):1–11. https://doi.org/10.1017/s0033291717001349.

40. Dalle Grave R, Eckhardt S, Calugi S, Le Grange D. A conceptual comparison of family-based treatment and enhanced cognitive behavior therapy in the treatment of adolescents with eating disorders. J Eat Disord. 2019;7(1):42. https://doi.org/10.1186/s40337-019-0275-x.

41. Dalle Grave R. Inpatient cognitive behavior therapy for severe eating disorders. Psychol Topic. 2010;19(2):323–40.

42. Calugi S, Dalle Grave R, Marchesini G. Longstanding underweight eating disorder: associated features and treatment outcome. Psychother Res. 2013;23(3):315–23. https://doi.org/10.1080/10503307.2012.717308.

Part II
Management of Complex Eating Disorder Cases

Chapter 4
General Strategies for the Management of Comorbidity in Eating Disorders

The term comorbidity was coined by Feinstein [1], who called it "any distinct clinical entity that has coexisted or that may occur during the clinical course of a patient who has the index disease under study" (pp. 456–7). However, this term has become frequently used in psychiatry to indicate not only the coexistence of a psychiatric diagnosis and a general medical one (e.g. major depression and type 2 diabetes) but also the coexistence of two or more psychiatric diagnoses (e.g. major depression, panic disorder and eating disorder) [2].

Issues related to the definition of comorbidity have important consequences for treatment. For example, the characteristics of depression are common in patients with eating disorders, but they may be evidence of coexisting clinical depression ("true comorbidity") or the direct consequence of eating disorder psychopathology ("spurious comorbidity"). In the first case, clinical depression should be treated directly, while in the second case the treatment of the eating disorder psychopathology should lead to remission of the depressive features.

However, comorbidity is a conceptually, clinically and psychometrically complex issue. The definition of comorbidity from a conceptual point of view refers to a situation in which "a distinct clinical entity develops during a disease" (e.g. when a patient with diabetes mellitus develops Parkinson's disease). In this case, there are two separate clinical entities, and comorbidity refers to a lifetime concept. In contrast, from a clinical point of view, the definition of comorbidity refers to a situation in which "two or more separate clinical entities coexist". In this case, the prevalence of comorbidity depends on the definition of the disorders in question (i.e. the diagnostic classification system and its rules). In the field of mental illness, where no specific biomarkers have been found so far, it is debatable whether these are indeed "distinct clinical entities" [2], or are simply artificial products of the current classification system. In fact, the diagnostic criteria described in the last edition of the DSM-5 [3] encourages the application of several psychiatric diagnoses in the same patient based on the symptoms presented. This could explain the current tendency to formulate, perhaps unnecessarily, more hypotheses than those necessary to

R. Dalle Grave et al., *Complex Cases and Comorbidity in Eating Disorders*, https://doi.org/10.1007/978-3-030-69341-1_4

explain a given phenomenon, when the initial, simplest ones would be sufficient, as per Occam's razor [4].

From a psychometric perspective the conceptualization of comorbidity has been called into question by recent evidence [5]. Under the theory of latent variables, which underlies the DSM-5 classification and has, until now, dominated the panorama of research into mental illness, the symptoms of mental disorders are conceptualized as the expression of a common latent entity. This theory postulates that there are underlying latent variables representing mental disorders that produce the specific symptoms which are experienced by individuals with these disorders. For example, major depressive disorder is a latent variable that determines a constellation of symptoms, such as depressed mood and anhedonia. In line with this model, comorbidity is due to the direct (bi)directional relationship between two or more latent variables. According to this model, if a latent variable causes the observable symptoms, this should assume that all the symptoms have a common cause, and are therefore unrelated to each other. Indeed, from a strictly psychometric point of view, if a single common cause (e.g. major depressive disorder) is responsible for the occurrence of a particular set of variables (i.e. symptoms of depression), then the potential association among these variables should be entirely explained by the presence of the common cause (i.e. major depressive disorder). However, this assumption is highly questionable, and clinicians, while adhering to the concept of the latent variable, at the same time recognize the direct relationships that exist between symptoms.

The complex network theory has recently been proposed to address these issues. This approach defines and analyses the relationships between symptoms without assuming from the outset that such relationships arise from a mental disorder as a common cause, but instead assessing how these symptoms might affect one another in a dynamic and random network [6, 7]. Within this theoretical and methodological framework, comorbidity is no longer seen as a direct relationship between two latent variables, but rather as a set of direct relationships between symptoms of different disorders. If mental disorders are closely connected networks of symptoms, there are no real boundaries between one disorder and another, and comorbidity can be represented by symptoms in common with multiple disorders, defined as "bridge symptoms" [5].

4.1   Epidemiological Data on Comorbidity in Eating Disorders

A narrative review of European studies concluded that more than 70% of people with eating disorders receive a diagnosis of at least one psychiatric comorbidity [8]. The most frequently mental illnesses reported as coexisting are anxiety disorders (>50%), mood disorders (>40%), self-harm (>20%) and substance use disorders (>10%). The lifetime occurrence of obsessions and compulsions also seems to be very frequent, and has been found to be present in about 70% of cases of anorexia nervosa [9]. An aggregation has also been discerned between autism spectrum disorders in probands with anorexia nervosa and their relatives [10]. Finally, there is some evidence of an association between attention-deficit hyperactivity disorder and eating disorders [11].

It should be noted, however, that data from the studies conducted to date present a wide variability in the rate of psychiatric comorbidity in eating disorders. For example, a lifetime history of an anxiety disorder has been reported in as few as 25% to as many as 75% of cases [12]. This wide range inevitably casts significant doubts on the reliability of these observations.

An even wider variability, ranging from 27% to 93%, has been reported on the prevalence of coexisting personality disorders [13]. Anorexia nervosa has been most frequently associated with an avoidant personality disorder—Cluster C (anxious or fearful disorders), while bulimia nervosa is more often seen in conjunction with Cluster B (dramatic, emotional or erratic disorders) [14]. However, a recent meta-analysis, which found a 53% prevalence of personality disorders in patients with any type of eating disorder, as compared to 9% in healthy controls, did not find any statistically significant differences in the total prevalence of personality disorders or in the various clusters of personality disorders between anorexia nervosa (49%) and bulimia nervosa (54%), except for obsessive-compulsive personality disorder, which was more prevalent in anorexia nervosa (23%) than in bulimia nervosa (12%) [15].

4.2 Methodological Problems with Studies Assessing Comorbidity in Eating Disorders

Studies that have assessed comorbidity in eating disorders suffer from serious methodological flaws that explain the embarrassing wide variability in the results reported. In summary, the main methodological problems with the research conducted to date are as follows:

- *Chronological onset*: a distinction has not always been made as to whether the comorbid disorder occurred before or after an eating disorder.
- *Small sample size*: the samples evaluated were mostly small, and as a result studies have often had statistical power too low for reliable conclusions to be drawn.
- *Clinical samples*: the majority of studies have assessed comorbidity in clinical samples, in which the prevalence of psychiatric comorbidity is likely to be overestimated (as compared to non-clinical samples).
- *Sample composition*: studies have included samples with different proportions of eating disorder diagnostic categories.
- *Heterogeneous diagnostic tools:* a wide variety of heterogeneous diagnostic interviews and self-administered questionnaires have been used to assess comorbidity.

- *Limited use of control groups*: studies rarely included age- and sex-matched controls.
- *No assessment of the secondary effects of the eating disorder psychopathology*: studies seldom assessed whether the comorbidity features were, in fact, secondary to the eating disorder psychopathology.
- *Diagnosis performed by researchers or clinicians:* the prevalence of comorbidity may vary if the diagnosis has been made by researchers using standardized tools as opposed to clinicians who do not.

In addition, there are numerous issues that complicate the interpretation of personality disorder data in patients with eating disorders [13]. In particular, it is difficult to assess the true personality of patients with an eating disorder because this is dramatically influenced by the psychopathology of the eating disorder itself and the consequences of undereating and low weight, i.e. starvation symptoms (see Chap. 2) [16]. Moreover, it is risky to make a diagnosis of coexisting personality disorders because many patients with eating disorders, in whom eating disorder onset occurs at a young age, have not actually experienced periods free from the presence of the eating disorder [17].

4.3   Comorbidity or Complex Cases?

The use of the term "comorbidity" to indicate the coexistence of two or more psychiatric diagnoses is considered hazardous by some authors because, in most cases, it is unclear whether concurrent diagnoses reflect the presence of distinct clinical entities or instead refer to multiple manifestations of a single clinical entity [2]. It is a fact that the diagnosis of multiple coexisting psychiatric diagnoses has become more frequent. This is partly the consequence of the use of standardized diagnostic interviews, which help to identify several clinical aspects that in the past have remained unnoticed after the main diagnosis, but it is also likely the consequence of the current DSM-5 classification system for at least four main reasons [2]:

1. The use of the implicit rule that the same symptom should not appear in more than one disorder (e.g. the symptom of anxiety should not appear in the diagnostic criteria of major depression, although people with depression often have symptoms of anxiety);
2. The proliferation of new psychiatric diagnostic categories;
3. The limited use of hierarchical diagnostic categories;
4. The use of operational criteria rather than criteria based on clinical descriptions to make the diagnosis.

The artificial division of complex clinical conditions into small "comorbidities" has the negative effects of preventing a more holistic approach to the person, and fostering the unjustified use of multiple drugs to treat individual pieces of a larger and more complex clinical picture. For this reason, we think that for eating disorders it seems more appropriate and clinically useful to talk about "complex cases" rather than comorbidity. Indeed, the notion that there is only a subset of "complex cases" cannot be applied to eating disorders [17], as in fact almost all patients with eating disorders can be considered complex cases. As described above, most meet the diagnostic criteria for one or more DSM-5 mental disorders, particularly clinical depression, anxiety disorders and substance use disorders, and many are diagnosed as having a personality disorder. Physical complications are common, and many patients have one or more coexisting and interacting medical diseases. Interpersonal difficulties are almost always present, and the enduring persistence of the disorder can have a strong negative impact on the development and interpersonal functioning of the individual. All these features indicate that complexity is the norm rather than the exception in patients with eating disorders [17].

4.4 CBT-E's Pragmatic Approach to Complex Cases

Given the difficulties associated with the definition of comorbidity, and in accordance with the CBT-E guidelines [18], we suggest taking a pragmatic approach to the assessment and management of the psychiatric and general medical problems that coexist with eating disorder. In short, comorbidities should be recognized, but only assessed for treatment when significant and having clinical implications.

Hence, we find it clinically useful to divide comorbidity into three main groups [18]:

- *Disorders that do not interfere with the treatment of eating disorders and that probably respond to it.* These disorders should be recognized, monitored and reassessed during treatment, but are not given special attention. Examples are as follows:

  - Secondary clinical depression (attributable to an eating disorder)
  - Social anxiety (attributable to an eating disorder)
  - Malnutrition
  - Unstable type 1 diabetes

- *Disorders that do not interfere with the treatment of eating disorders but do not respond to it.* These disorders must be recognized, and a decision made on when to address them. As a general rule, it is advisable to treat such disorders before or after the eating disorder psychopathology, especially if they need to be managed via psychological treatments. Examples are as follows:

  - Post-traumatic stress disorder, including reported sexual abuse
  - Obsessive-compulsive disorder (which may be treated using selective serotonin reuptake inhibitors (SSRIs) during CBT-E for the eating disorder)
  - Obesity

- *Disorders that interfere with the treatment of eating disorders.* These disorders need to be recognized and addressed before starting CBT-E. Examples are as follows:
  - Continuous substance misuse
  - Acute psychotic disorders
  - Clinical depression (not attributable to the eating disorder)

4.5   Multidisciplinary Management of Complex Cases

Given the prevalence of medical and psychopathological comorbidity in eating disorders, the assessment and management of such patients often necessitate a multidisciplinary approach, and therefore the involvement of multiple healthcare professionals. However, multidisciplinary teams have the tendency to adopt an "eclectic" approach, usually encompassing a wide range of medical, psychiatric, psychological and educational procedures derived from different, sometimes conflicting, theories. For example, a psychologist may deliver psychoanalytic psychotherapy while a dietitian relies on behavioural procedures at the same time as a psychiatrist and internist are assessing and treating the various comorbidities using different types of drugs. In other words, the members of the team follow the theory and practice they have learned in their studies, pursuing therapeutic objectives related to their professional role rather than those of the team as a whole.

While each of these individual approaches may have some merit and, to some extent, provide some benefit to patients, their co-administration inevitably entails numerous potential clinical disadvantages [19]:

- *High costs.* Treatments that routinely involve many professionals inevitably have high costs, which have a major impact on the national health service and/or families.
- *Nobody sees the complete clinical picture of the patient.* Patients' problems are inevitably broken down, discussed and addressed by different therapists.
- *Contradictory information.* Patients often receive contradictory information about their eating disorder, and the strategies and procedures needed to address it. This mixture of information inevitably creates confusion in patients and a sense of loss of control, compromising the effectiveness of individual treatments.
- *Unclear therapeutic boundaries.* Therapists may unwittingly encroach on the territory of another team member, generating further confusion in patients. For example, a dietitian, frustrated by the dietary difficulties shown by some patients, may provide a naive psychological interpretation of their ambivalence, effectively taking on the role of the psychologist.
- *Conflict between team members.* In this scenario, conflicts between team members are likely to arise, especially among clinicians who have different beliefs about how to treat eating disorder psychopathology and coexisting problems.

Friction between therapists may increase a patient's ambivalence towards change and thereby compromise the treatment outcome.

- *Difficulties in assessing the effectiveness and active elements of the treatment.* Without a shared protocol, it is almost impossible to assess the treatment effectiveness to the standards required by evidence-based medicine. Besides, without a unifying theory, it is almost impossible to understand what the active elements of the treatment are. As a consequence, it is very unlikely that a real improvement in the effectiveness of the treatment can occur.
- *Problems in disseminating the treatment.* The dissemination and replication of treatment strategies and procedures used in eclectic multidisciplinary approaches are very complex.

Moreover, we have often observed in our clinical practice patients who have experienced poor management of coexisting psychiatric and general medical problems by eclectic multidisciplinary teams not guided by a common theoretical model. Indeed, clearly spurious comorbidities, i.e. those in reality produced by the effects of eating disorder psychopathology and/or malnutrition, frequently receive a diagnosis of psychiatric and/or medical comorbidity, and are treated accordingly, often with improper cocktails of drugs. Comorbidities are even more likely to be diagnosed if patients are assessed by psychiatrists or physicians who are unfamiliar with the effects of eating disorder psychopathology and/or malnutrition, who tend to attribute the signs and symptoms of the consequences of eating disorder to comorbidity.

4.5.1 The Non-Eclectic CBT-E Multidisciplinary Team

To address the problems inherent in an eclectic multidisciplinary team described above, we have designed an adaptation of CBT-E suitable for application at three levels of care (outpatient, day-hospital and hospital), called *multistep* CBT-E (see Chap. 3, Sect. 3.4.5); it is designed to be delivered by a "non-eclectic" multidisciplinary team whose members are fully trained in CBT-E. The multidisciplinary CBT-E team adopts four main strategies to ensure that all members of the team are aware of a patient's entire clinical picture and avoid providing contradictory advice [19].

1. *Therapist training.* All team members (i.e. physicians, psychiatrists, psychologists, dietitians and nurses) involved in the assessment and/or management of the patients in intensive settings (e.g. day-hospital or impatient) receive extensive training in CBT-E before joining the team. This ensures that while the therapists maintain their specific professional roles, they all share the same philosophy (cognitive behaviour theory and therapy) and therefore use a similar language with patients. Thus, after the assessment and preparation sessions, in which an experienced doctor from the team is involved in assessing whether the potential comorbidities associated with an eating disorder are real or spurious, CBT-E can

be administered by either a single therapist (i.e. outpatient CBT-E) or by the non-eclectic multidisciplinary team (i.e. intensive outpatient CBT-E and inpatient CBT-E). Although under this system most outpatient cases only require the intervention of a single team member, generally the CBT psychologist, periodic examination by a team psychiatrist and/or physician can be integrated without interrupting the general flow of the treatment. Indeed, other specialists may be needed to treat patients with coexisting psychiatric disorders (e.g. clinical depression), medical conditions (e.g. obesity, type 1 or type 2 diabetes), or complications associated with their low weight and/or purging, but these interventions are always agreed to with the therapist who administers CBT-E following the pragmatic guidelines described in this chapter. In addition, regular advice from a dietitian trained in CBT-E can be indicated and supplemented in patients with obesity (BMI ≥30.0) or severely low body weight (BMI <16.0), or in those who want to continue to follow a vegetarian or vegan diet for ethical or religious reasons. Table 4.1 provides some tips for building a multidisciplinary CBT-E team [19].

Table 4.1 Practical advice on building a multidisciplinary CBT-E team

1.	Select, if possible, open-minded young therapists who are not committed to other theories and therapeutic practices. Strong alternative influences may be dangerous because they may cause a therapist to deviate too far from the treatment guidelines.
2.	Train all therapists (psychologists, dietitians, psychiatrists, physicians and nurses) in CBT-E and in the team approach before they start to see patients.[a] Neither universities nor psychotherapy schools (even CBT-based) tend to prepare therapists in both CBT-E and teamwork.
3.	Monitor therapist fidelity and consistency by adopting the following procedures: • Planning a weekly peer-supervised meeting between therapists to discuss clinical work freely and at length • Asking the therapists to record individual sessions and encouraging them to listen to selected recordings of each others' treatment sessions • Asking the therapists to provide evidence of the topics covered in each session as an integral part of medical record-keeping • Providing therapists with a written treatment protocol to implement • Introducing new procedures and strategies only when mutually agreed upon
4.	Provide procedures to improve the team approach, including but not limited to: • Maintaining the highest standard of professional knowhow in the team, with regular group updates on eating disorder literature • Pooling knowledge to be gained in the field with all team members • Helping other team members to resolve problems implementing CBT-E • Never criticizing other team members (in the presence of either the patient or the other team members) • Organizing weekly team meetings to set out the professional tasks of each member in detail, address any difficulties raised by the implementation of the treatment, and integrate new strategies and procedures

[a]The First Certificate of Professional Training in Eating Disorders and Obesity is an annual advanced training diploma awarded following a course designed to train specialists from different disciplines (physicians, psychologists, dietitians and nutritionists) in the cognitive behaviour theory and therapy of eating disorders and obesity, and to work as part of a non-eclectic multidisciplinary team. In Italy, more than 500 clinicians have participated in this course to date

2. *Role definition and coordination.* To take advantage of the flexibility of this unified multidisciplinary approach, it is essential that the therapeutic roles within the team are well defined and coordinated. For example, in intensive outpatient CBT-E and inpatient CBT-E, the role of the dietitian is to address the modification of eating habits and weight, while the psychologist tackles body image, events and mood changes influencing eating and any additional maintenance processes, and the physician oversees the physical health of patients and prescription of drugs. In addition, in the inpatient treatment, the nurse takes care of the administration of medications and assists patients during weighing and in the management of daily difficulties. Other professionals may be recruited, such as educators to help younger patients carry out schoolwork and other educational activities, and physiotherapists to manage physical rehabilitation sessions, but are also fully trained in CBT-E and seamlessly integrated into the non-eclectic multidisciplinary team.

3. *Weekly review meeting.* In intensive care settings, weekly review sessions are organized featuring the input of both the patient and all their therapists (round table). In this meeting, the patient's progress is reviewed, and the various elements of the treatment and their relationship to one another are discussed. This enables all team members to form a complete picture of the patient's eating problem, and gives the patient a sense of empowerment, at the same time obviating the risk of mixed messages arising.

4. *Personal formulation.* This is a visual representation of the processes that appear to be maintaining the patient's eating disorder (see Chap. 3, Sect. 3.4.2). It is built collaboratively with the patient, and can be used as a guide to integrating each team member's contribution to the treatment. This will ensure that no therapist oversteps the boundaries of his or her professional role, and that the patient receives comprehensive and coherent individualized treatment.

References

1. Feinstein AR. The pre-therapeutic classification of co-morbidity in chronic disease. J Chronic Dis. 1970;23(7):455–68. https://doi.org/10.1016/0021-9681(70)90054-8.
2. Maj M. "Psychiatric comorbidity": an artefact of current diagnostic systems? Br J Psychiatry. 2005;186:182–4. https://doi.org/10.1192/bjp.186.3.182.
3. American Psychiatric Association. Diagnostic and statistical manual of mental disorders, (DSM-5). Arlington: American Psychiatric Publishing; 2013.
4. Gutiérrez E, Carrera O. Anorexia nervosa treatments and Occam's razor. Psychol Med. 2018;48(8):1390–1. https://doi.org/10.1017/s0033291717003944.
5. Cramer AO, Waldorp LJ, van der Maas HL, Borsboom D. Comorbidity: a network perspective. Behav Brain Sci. 2010;33(2–3):137–50; discussion 50-93. https://doi.org/10.1017/s0140525x09991567.
6. Borsboom D. Psychometric perspectives on diagnostic systems. J Clin Psychol. 2008;64(9):1089–108. https://doi.org/10.1002/jclp.20503.
7. van der Maas HL, Dolan CV, Grasman RP, Wicherts JM, Huizenga HM, Raijmakers ME. A dynamical model of general intelligence: the positive manifold of intelligence by mutualism. Psychol Rev. 2006;113(4):842–61. https://doi.org/10.1037/0033-295x.113.4.842.

8. Keski-Rahkonen A, Mustelin L. Epidemiology of eating disorders in Europe: prevalence, incidence, comorbidity, course, consequences, and risk factors. Curr Opin Psychiatry. 2016;29(6):340–5. https://doi.org/10.1097/yco.0000000000000278.

9. Halmi KA, Sunday SR, Klump KL, Strober M, Leckman JF, Fichter M, et al. Obsessions and compulsions in anorexia nervosa subtypes. Int J Eat Disord. 2003;33(3):308–19. https://doi.org/10.1002/eat.10138.

10. Koch SV, Larsen JT, Mouridsen SE, Bentz M, Petersen L, Bulik C, et al. Autism spectrum disorder in individuals with anorexia nervosa and in their first- and second-degree relatives: Danish nationwide register-based cohort-study. Br J Psychiatry. 2015;206(5):401–7. https://doi.org/10.1192/bjp.bp.114.153221.

11. Sala L, Martinotti G, Carenti ML, Romo L, Oumaya M, Pham-Scottez A, et al. Attention-deficit/hyperactivity disorder symptoms and psychological comorbidity in eating disorder patients. Eat Weight Disord. 2018;23(4):513–9. https://doi.org/10.1007/s40519-017-0395-8.

12. Swinbourne JM, Touyz SW. The co-morbidity of eating disorders and anxiety disorders: a review. Eur Eat Disord Rev. 2007;15(4):253–74. https://doi.org/10.1002/erv.784.

13. Vitousek K, Manke F. Personality variables and disorders in anorexia nervosa and bulimia nervosa. J Abnorm Psychol. 1994;103(1):137–47. https://doi.org/10.1037//0021-843x.103.1.137.

14. Cassin SE, von Ranson KM. Personality and eating disorders: a decade in review. Clin Psychol Rev. 2005;25(7):895–916. https://doi.org/10.1016/j.cpr.2005.04.012.

15. Martinussen M, Friborg O, Schmierer P, Kaiser S, Overgard KT, Neunhoeffer AL, et al. The comorbidity of personality disorders in eating disorders: a meta-analysis. Eat Weight Disord. 2017;22(2):201–9. https://doi.org/10.1007/s40519-016-0345-x.

16. Garner DM, Dalle Grave R. Terapia cognitivo comportamentale dei disturbi dell'alimentazione. Verona: Positive Press; 1999.

17. Fairburn CG. Cognitive behavior therapy and eating disorders. New York: Guilford Press; 2008.

18. Fairburn CG, Cooper Z, Waller D. Complex cases and comorbidity. In: Fairburn CG, editor. Cognitive behavior therapy and eating disorders. New York: Guilford Press; 2008.

19. Dalle Grave R. Multistep cognitive behavioral therapy for eating disorders: theory, practice, and clinical cases. New York: Jason Aronson; 2013.

Chapter 5
Coexisting Psychological Problems

A series of systematic clinical observations on patients who showed a poor response to CBT for bulimia nervosa—a treatment specifically designed to address only the eating disorder psychopathology—revealed that there was a group of patients with one or more additional psychological problems that had interfered with the response to treatment [1]. These psychological problems were identified as clinical perfectionism, core low self-esteem, marked interpersonal difficulties, and mood intolerance, and the treatment was adapted in order to treat these conditions alongside the eating disorder. The result of this was the "broad" form of CBT-E (see Chap. 3, Sect. 3.4.3), which includes specific modules to address each of these "external" processes, which through different mechanisms contribute to maintaining the eating disorder psychopathology and therefore hinder change [1].

The broad form of CBT-E should be reserved for about 25–30% patients in whom one or more external psychological problems exhibit all of the following three characteristics [2]: (i) they are pronounced, (ii) appear to maintain the eating disorder psychopathology, and (iii) seem to impede response to treatment. As a general guideline, in underweight patients, broad CBT-E is used only if there is clear evidence that the external maintenance process is interfering with weight regain. In fact, in many patients it is often observed that the normalization of body weight and the gradual removal of the eating disorder psychopathology produce an improvement in self-esteem and interpersonal difficulties and, in some cases, also in perfectionist attitudes and the ability to regulate emotions. If more than one external mechanism is identified, we suggest addressing the one that seems to be contributing most to the maintenance of the eating disorder.

The decision on whether or not to use the broad form of CBT-E is usually taken during one or two review sessions after 4 weeks from the start of the treatment in patients who are not underweight, or in one of the later review sessions in underweight patients. Having concluded that broad CBT-E is indicated, the subsequent individual CBT-E sessions have two main aims [3]:

1. To address the specific maintenance processes of eating disorder psychopathology with the focused form of CBT-E;
2. To address the identified external process using the broad CBT-E module(s).

Since the two aims are allocated the same time within the session, this results in less time being available to address the eating disorder psychopathology. For this reason, we suggest increasing the standard length of the treatment by about 10 sessions (i.e. from 20 to 30 sessions in not underweight patients, and from 30–40 sessions to 40–50 sessions in underweight patients) so that more time can be devoted to addressing the external psychological process(es).

5.1 Clinical Perfectionism

Traits of perfectionism are often evident in people with eating disorders and may even be present before the onset of the disorder itself. It is not clear whether they affect the outcome of the treatment, but at the extreme end of this spectrum is what is called "clinical perfectionism", a condition in which perfectionism is so pronounced that the person's life is significantly damaged. Clinical perfectionism seems to maintain the eating disorder psychopathology and negatively interfere with the treatment [4], and should therefore be addressed in conjunction with the eating disorder psychopathology.

5.1.1 Characteristics of Clinical Perfectionism

It has been proposed that the core psychopathology of clinical perfectionism is the "overvaluation of achieving (and striving to achieve) personally demanding standards in areas of life valued as important, despite adverse consequences" [4]. According to this definition, clinical perfectionism is a psychopathology equivalent to the core eating disorder psychopathology (i.e. the overvaluation of shape, weight and eating and their control—see Chap. 2) as it is a dysfunctional scheme of self-evaluation. Like the overvaluation of shape, weight, eating and their control, the core psychopathology of clinical perfectionism has various harmful expressions that maintain the overvaluation of achieving (Fig. 5.1).

When clinical perfectionism coexists with an eating disorder, the demanding standards are also applied to shape, weight, eating and their control. Consequently, the diet and other features of the eating disorder psychopathology (e.g. excessive exercising and body checking) are intensified (Fig. 5.2). Furthermore, the tenacity in pursuing these standards increases, and there is a reluctance to change. In this way, the psychopathology of clinical perfectionism intensifies the eating disorder psychopathology and creates an obstacle to change.

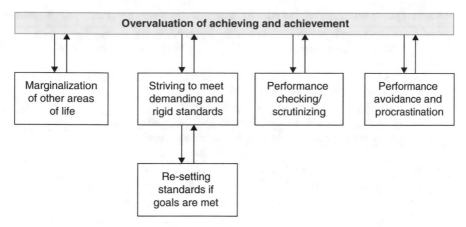

Fig. 5.1 Formulation of an adult patient with an eating disorder featuring overvaluation of achieving and achievement. Reproduced with permission from the Online Training Programme in CBT-E, CREDO Oxford, 2017

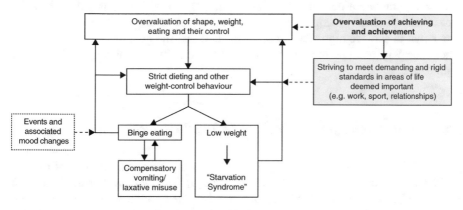

Fig. 5.2 The interaction between clinical perfectionism and eating-disorder psychopathology. Reproduced with permission from the Online Training Programme in CBT-E, CREDO Oxford, 2017

5.1.2   Assessing for the Presence of Clinical Perfectionism

Clinical perfectionism should be suspected if a patient fills in their monitoring records in an excessively detailed way, adopts dietary rules that are particularly extreme and rigid, and slows down the treatment by getting lost in the details of the procedures to apply. Other common clues are if a patient dedicates the majority of the day studying or doing sport, despite significant others' advice to reduce their commitment to this activity. In these cases, the therapist should ask a series of questions (Table 5.1) that may help to discern whether clinical perfectionism may coexist with the eating disorder psychopathology.

If clinical perfectionism is pronounced, appears to maintain the eating disorder psychopathology, and hinder response to treatment, we explain the nature of its

Table 5.1 Questions that can help the clinician understand if a patient has clinical perfectionism

Some people with an eating problem might be described as "perfectionists" because they set high standards and are constantly striving to achieve them. Would this describe you? What do others say about you?

- Do you set yourself higher standards than others? What do others think? In which areas of life do you set high standards (school, work, sport, music, etc.)?
- How important is it for you to work hard and do well?
- Do you spend a lot of time thinking about the goals you want to achieve?
- If you reach one of your goals, do you immediately set a higher one?
- Do you repeatedly check your performance and compare it to that of others?
- Are you afraid of not being able to achieve your goals?
- Do you avoid doing things for fear that your performance will not be enough good?
- Do you tend to judge yourself on the effort you put into trying to reach your goals and their achievement?

psychopathology, its expressions, the impairment it causes (e.g. worsening of performance, marginalization of other aspects of life) and how it maintains the eating disorder, drawing a personal formulation similar to that shown in Fig. 5.2. If the patient has difficulty recognizing clinical perfectionism as a problem, considering it essential to achieve high standards, we explain that the goal of the treatment is to help them to achieve the same results but with different and more functional strategies.

5.1.3 Strategies for Addressing Clinical Perfectionism

Clinical perfectionism is treated by CBT-E using a strategy similar to that used to address the overvaluation of shape and weight [3]. The two psychopathologies are discussed more or less in tandem, but it is advisable to address body image a few weeks before. This is because the clinical perfectionism module builds on the understanding acquired by patients when addressing body image.

The strategy used to address clinical perfectionism involves the application of the following procedures, which have been described in detail in previous publications [2–6]:

- Identifying the overvaluation of achieving and its consequences (see above).
- Enhancing the importance of other domains of life. Patients are encouraged to choose activities in which performance is not easily quantified (e.g. reading novels/newspaper, listening to music, staying in touch with friends).
- Addressing perfectionist standards and striving. The goals of treatment are to modify the patient's standards to make them less demanding and flexible rather than rigid.
- Addressing performance checking (i.e. repeated assessment of performance, generally focused on perceived shortcomings). Behaviours to address are

checking personal performance, comparison making (comparing personal performance with that of others), and reassurance checking (asking others about
one's performance).
- Addressing performance/avoidance. Behaviours to address are avoidance of performance self-assessment and external performance testing (school tests, sports
competitions, social events, singing in front of others, and so on).
- Exploring the origins of the overvaluation. Looking for events or circumstances
that might have sensitized the patients to performance issues.
- Dealing with setbacks. Patients are helped to learn to regulate their clinical perfectionism mindset by learning how to do the following three things: (i) identifying setback triggers, (ii) recognizing the first signs that the perfectionism mindset
has returned, and (iii) displacing the mindset.
- Ending well. Patients are helped to identify residual problems and devise a specific perfectionism-oriented maintenance plan to address residual perfectionist
attitudes and behaviours and prevent relapse.

Vignette
The patient is a 20-year-old woman attending literature classes at the university. She
is an only child, both parents are lawyers, and her mother was mayor of the small
town in which they live. The patient reported that she had been a quiet and reserved
child, very proud of her parents, who she admired for what they did. Indeed, her
family is very prominent in the town, widely recognized for their social and political
achievements.

At secondary school, the patient performed very well and had the feeling that
others expected precisely that from her. In any case, she liked to be good at school
and worked hard to achieve excellent grades. However, at high school she found that
she needed to work harder, and felt greater pressure to compete with her classmates.
She began to have difficulties, especially in Greek and Latin, and realized that she
was no longer the best in the class. Indeed, two classmates got higher marks than her
in all subjects. These were twin sisters who were both very thin and who openly
flaunted their slim figures and skills in front of others. The patient began to intensify
her efforts to compete, studying from when she returned home from school until
dinner time without ever stopping. She would then study for a couple of hours after
dinner, and often got up very early in the morning (around 5:30) to go over what she
had learned. She lost all interest in social relationships, which had previously been
good albeit limited, and focused entirely on her school performance.

By the age of 16, her studies had become so important (her goal was to get top
marks in all subjects) that she began to skip snacks, eating only a quick lunch and
dinner so as not to "waste time", and to keep from putting on weight—a feeling that
she felt would take her focus away from studying. In this period she was very satisfied with herself. Indeed, she achieved excellent results at school, and at the same
time she liked her new body shape, after having lost 3 kg (from 56 to 53 kg).
Moreover, she received positive comments about her body shape from several classmates (even the twins). However, she became progressively more concerned about
food and eating, and her eating rules became rigid and extreme.

In the following years, she avoided eating several food types (e.g. desserts, pasta and carbs in general) and eschewed all occasions for social eating, continuing to study for many hours every day. Her body weight dropped to 48 kg, and her preoccupation with her shape, weight and eating control became extreme. Despite this, she still felt that everything was fine, and that she could keep her life under perfect control.

Later, however, she sought medical advice because she was having difficulties at university. Her concentration was poor, and she had actively avoided taking exams because she was unable to memorize what she was reading, despite having intensified the hours dedicated to her studies. She felt very tired, frustrated and a failure. Her body weight was 42.4 kg (BMI 15.4), but, despite her low weight, she had an extreme fear of weight gain and had adopted extreme dietary restriction.

The patient was immediately engaged in CBT-E and, at the end of Step One, decided to address weight gain in order to recover her strength and concentration. With the initial weight regain she achieved during Step Two of the treatment, the patient felt better and reported an improvement in her concentration. She reached a body weight of 48 kg (BMI 17.4), but she still avoided taking university exams as she felt insufficiently prepared. She also developed a belief that continuing to regain weight was not necessary. In fact, she reported that this would require an increase in the amount of food she would need to eat, which would probably intensify her digestive difficulties and, as a consequence, impair her concentration during studies. Moreover, she thought that her thighs were already getting too big.

The patient gradually restarted her usual efforts to study, waking up at 5 am, reading a paragraph and taking notes, then reading another one and taking notes again, until she had finished each textbook. Once she had arranged her notes, she would make outlines of them, then underline the important points in the outlines. Before going to bed at 11:30 pm, she reviewed everything she had studied, trying to memorize the highlights. When she realized she was unable to remember something, she would start the process again until she was able to remember everything perfectly by heart. Sometimes this process lasted until 3:00 am. She avoided taking exams at the university, but reported going to observe her classmates' oral exams and noting down all the questions asked by the professors. At home, she would try to answer these questions and, when she had difficulty, criticized herself and spent the following days reviewing the subjects raised by the questions.

During one of the review sessions in Step Two, the therapist, having noted that her clinical perfectionism was extreme, hindering the treatment and maintaining the eating disorder psychopathology, raised the possibility of addressing it as part of the treatment. The patient recognized that she had the problem of clinical perfectionism, which in her was expressed in two main domains, namely the achievement of extremely high standards at university, and control of weight, shape and eating. Shared processes identified in these two domains were repeated performance checking and body checking, striving to study and follow dietary rules, avoiding tests and body exposure, and resetting goals if her standards were met. She also agreed that her system of self-evaluation was counterproductive because it impaired both her performance at university and her physical and psychosocial well-being. In Step Two, albeit with difficulty, she gradually addressed all the maintenance mechanisms in her personal formulation, implementing the CBT-E body image, dietary restraint and clinical perfectionism modules, and reaching a low-normal body weight (BMI 19.1). At the same time, the therapist helped her to develop new, performance-free domains of self-evaluation (e.g. listening to music, spending time with friends).

At the end of the treatment, the clinical perfectionism was still evident, but she allowed herself greater flexibility in terms of her diet, and had interrupted her dysfunctional checking and avoidance. She was now devoting less time to her studies (not studying after dinner) and had taken and passed two exams. Finally, the introduction of performance-free activities was enabling her to spend some free time with two friends from university.

5.2   Core Low Self-Esteem

Most people with eating disorders have low self-esteem, being highly self-critical as a result of their perceived failure to attain their goals of controlling shape, weight, and eating—a form of negative self-evaluation that may be termed "secondary self-criticism." This aspect of negative self-evaluation does not need to be addressed by the treatment because it generally does not obstruct the change, and improves when the eating disorder is successfully treated. There is, however, a subgroup of patients who have extremely low self-esteem or "core low self-esteem", which maintains the eating disorder and obstructs change [1]. In such cases, the chance of treatment success is poor [7] unless low self-esteem is directly addressed.

5.2.1   Characteristics of Core Low Self-Esteem

Core low self-esteem is defined as an unconditional and pervasive negative view of self-worth which is long-lasting, largely independent of current circumstances and performance, and not explained by the presence of clinical depression. This negative self-evaluation is autonomous and, therefore, minimally affected by changes in the state of the eating disorder. People with core low self-esteem believe that they have little or no value as a person, and describe themselves as "worthless", "useless", "stupid", "unlovable", "a failure" [2].

When core low self-esteem coexists with the eating disorder psychopathology, it obstructs the change through two main processes [3]: (i) the patients see little or no prospect of recovery as a result of the unconditional and pervasive nature of their negative view of themselves, and (ii) the low self-esteem leads them to strive especially hard to control their shape, weight and eating to assuage their sense of worthlessness (Fig. 5.3).

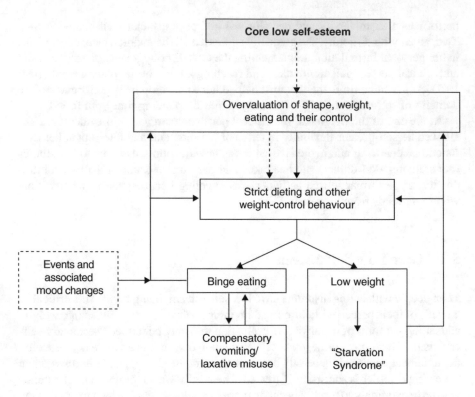

Fig. 5.3 The interaction between clinical core low self-esteem and the eating-disorder psychopathology. Reproduced with permission from the Online Training Programme in CBT-E, CREDO Oxford, 2017

5.2.2   Assessing for Core Low Self-Esteem

It is crucial to distinguish secondary self-criticism from core low self-esteem [2]:

1. *Secondary self-criticism* is conditional on current performance in valued areas of life and fluctuates (i.e. the patient is not constantly self-critical). People with eating disorders and secondary self-criticism do not consider themselves a failure as a person and do not view themselves in globally negative terms.
2. *Core low self-esteem* is characterized by an unconditionally negative view of self not influenced by specific aspects of performance. People with eating disorders and core low self-esteem have a negative overall view of their self-worth, and an inability to distance from a self-critical stance (i.e. a person's identity). They also tend to make negative comparisons with others.

   Other specific features of core low self-esteem are the presence of pronounced negative cognitive processing biases, such as a negative vision of the future and the belief in the impossibility to change. These not only obstruct the treatment, but core low self-esteem itself is a risk factor for the development of anorexia nervosa and bulimia nervosa [8, 9]. As it is longstanding, it is difficult to detect its onset, and it is also problematic to identify core low self-esteem when the patients have coexisting clinical depression. In this case, we suggest addressing clinical depression first (see Chap. 6, Sect. 6.1) and reassessing self-esteem afterwards.

5.2.3   Strategies for Addressing Core Low Self-Esteem

Core low self-esteem is addressed by CBT-E in two ways: (i) directly, with targeted cognitive behaviour procedures; and (ii) indirectly, by enhancing patients' interpersonal functioning (see Sect. 5.3). In general, if a patient displays evident cognitive biases, we use the direct method, while we opt for indirect methods when it seems feasible for a patient to create a network of positive interpersonal relationships. In the latter case, we explain to patients that the best way of improving their self-esteem would be to enhance the quality of their relationships.

The strategy used to address core low self-esteem directly involves the application of the following procedures, which have been described in detail in previous publications [2, 3, 10]:

- *Personalized education.* Patients are first educated on the main cognitive mechanisms maintaining their core low self-esteem, and how they interact with the eating disorder psychopathology (Fig. 5.4).
- *Addressing cognitive bias.* One or more of the following cognitive biases are addressed using conventional cognitive behavioural procedures:
  - Discounting positive qualities.
  - Selective attention (i.e. looking selectively for failure and finding it).
  - Double standards (i.e. having one set of [harsh] standards for judging themselves, and another [more lenient] set for others).
  - Overgeneralization (i.e. viewing any instance of not succeeding as a failure, and then generalizing from such failures to being "a failure" in general).
  - Dichotomous appraisals of self-worth (i.e. assessing themselves in all-or-nothing terms—"If I am not always strong, I must be a weak person").

- *Addressing problematic rules.* These are "rules of life" [11] that people with core low self-esteem use to cope with their negative core beliefs (i.e. "I need to be good at… to be worth something"). The problematic aspect of these rules is that, since they are rigid and extreme, they are inevitably broken, and this, consequently, leads the person with core low self-esteem to confirm their negative core self-belief.
- *Exploring the origins of the core low self-esteem*
- *Arriving at a balanced view of self-worth*

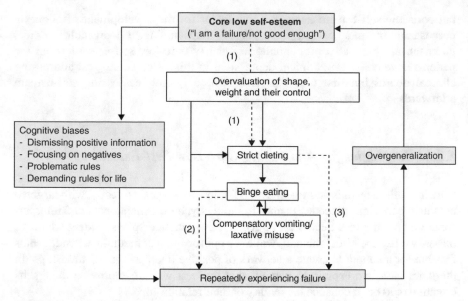

Fig. 5.4 Formulation showing how the specific expressions of core low self-esteem maintain the eating-disorder psychopathology
(1) The control of shape, weight, and eating is used to reduce feelings of worthlessness
(2) Binge eating is experienced as a failure and confirms negative self-belief
(3) Breaking a dietary rule is experienced as a failure and confirms negative self-belief
Reproduced with permission from the Online Training Programme in CBT-E, CREDO Oxford, 2017

Vignette

The patient is a 25-year-old woman and is preparing her university dissertation in Philosophy. She comes from a middle-class family; her father is a freelance professional and her mother a high-school teacher. The mother reported that the patient had been shy and introverted since she was a child, and has always had difficulty in creating friendships, always standing to the side and being easily ignored by others. She had always performed well at school, but invariably felt useless, despite her excellent grades.

At middle school she began to feel unsatisfied with the shape of her body, and at the age of 13 started a diet to lose weight. She thought that by losing weight she would feel better about herself, and be more accepted by others. Indeed, she had always felt inadequate in social situations, and not up to par. Moreover, she despised herself for this.

The dietary restriction and the consequent weight loss made her feel more in control. However, she continued to feel inadequate, her relationship with her friends (who relied on her for help with their homework) did not change, and her perceptions of being worthless remained unaffected. After a few months, the dietary restriction was recurrently interrupted by binge-eating episodes followed by self-induced vomiting. The binge-eating and vomiting episodes increased her sense of inadequacy. She often scolded herself for being useless as she was unable to control even her diet; she felt increasingly incapable and had come to hate herself. The alternation of dietary restraint, binge-eating and self-induced vomiting continued throughout her high school and university years, when her body weight remained stable at around 60–62 kg (BMI 22.0).

In recent months, however, the frequency of the patient's binge-eating and self-induced vomiting episodes had increased, and she was having some difficulty communicating with her dissertation supervisor. She had asked for a dissertation topic a few months earlier and, after the professor had given her a topic, started doing bibliographic research and writing, never asking for help or support. Indeed, she was afraid of appearing stupid if she asked for help because her rule was that a good student must be able to write a dissertation on their own. The professor, after having reviewed her draft dissertation, explicitly told her that she had not addressed the topic well and should focus more on its purpose. This comment threw the patient into utter despair, making her feel like a failure and unable to move forward with her dissertation.

At the first assessment and preparation session, the patient appeared very intimidated—she never looked the therapist in the eye, and reported judging herself as inadequate as a person and unable to keep control over eating. She expressed a desire to start a psychological treatment, but did not think she would be able to overcome her eating disorder.

Over the course of CBT-E Stage One, with the application of the regular eating procedure,[1] the frequency of binge-eating episodes reduced. Nonetheless, the patient was not always able to comply with regular eating, skipping several meals and making binge-eating more likely. In her monitoring records she wrote the following comments: "I hate myself; I am incapable of doing anything"; "I am a nobody and I don't deserve to eat"; "I will never be able to do anything in life if I am not even able to control my eating"; and "I am fat and ugly". She noted that these feelings of inadequacy grew stronger when she was working on her dissertation.

During a review session in Stage Two, the therapist discussed with the patient the evidence that core low self-esteem seemed to be hindering her treatment and contributing to the maintenance of her eating disorder, and that it should therefore be addressed. The patient agreed to this proposal, and half of the sessions in Stage Three were dedicated to tackling core low self-esteem, in addition to the usual procedures for addressing her eating disorder psychopathology. The therapist provided education about the cognitive biases that seemed to be maintaining the patient's low self-esteem, and encouraged her to monitor them in real time. This helped the patient recognize that the most prominent cognitive biases she had were discounting positive qualities ("I have no positive qualities"), selective attention to minor mistakes (labelled as "failures"), and overgeneralization ("I am a failure"). The

---

[1] The CBT-E regular eating procedure has two components: (i) eating three meals and two snacks every day; and (ii) not eating between meals and planned snacks.

therapist helped her to identify and correct these cognitive biases in real time, and encouraged her to focus on and accept her positive experiences. The patient was also encouraged to ask advice from her supervisor on how to better proceed with her dissertation in order to test the effect of breaking her rule of never asking for help (based on her assumption that "If I ask for help, the other will think that I am useless"). To her surprise, the professor was very kind and supported her work on her dissertation. This work gradually helped the patient to question her negative belief about herself, and start to believe that it would be possible to overcome her eating disorder. She therefore became more active in addressing dietary restraint and negative body image, and by the end of the treatment she had only a moderate preoccupation with shape and weight, and sporadic binge-eating episodes in the premenstrual phase. She also recognized that her view of being worthless and a failure was dysfunctional, and began, albeit with much difficulty, to address life by trying to accept her body weight and shape, and herself as a person.

5.3 Marked Interpersonal Difficulties

Interpersonal difficulties are common in people with eating disorders, but generally they resolve with improvement in the eating disorder psychopathology and do not interfere with treatment. For this reason, they often do not have to be directly addressed as CBT-E's proactive problem-solving procedure helps patients to successfully address most interpersonal problems associated with changes in eating. However, in a subgroup of patients with an eating disorder, marked interpersonal problems may maintain the patient's eating disorder and/or interfere with the implementation of treatment [3].

5.3.1 Characteristics of Marked Interpersonal Difficulties

In general, the interpersonal difficulties typically seen in patients with eating disorders can be divided into three main categories [2]: (i) social isolation and interpersonal functioning deficit, (ii) interpersonal conflicts, and (iii) role transitions. These interpersonal difficulties maintain the eating disorder and/or interfere with the implementation of the CBT-E causing one of the following consequences:

1. *Interpersonal turbulence.* When interpersonal difficulties hijack treatment sessions or interfere with the patients' compliance with homework between sessions.
2. *Interpersonal vacuum.* When an absence of relationships prevents patients from exploiting some aspects of treatment (such as developing new self-evaluation domains).

5.3.2 Assessing for Marked Interpersonal Difficulties

A strategy we use to identify relevant interpersonal areas is building an interpersonal history with patients [3]. As part of this task, we seek to identify any potentially problematic interpersonal events associated with the development and maintenance of the patient's eating disorder. Assessment of a patient's interpersonal history can help to elucidate whether interpersonal difficulties are contributing significantly to maintaining the eating disorder and/or are interfering with the implementation of treatment. In some cases, as described in Sect. 5.2.3, we address core low self-esteem by tackling interpersonal difficulties.

If the conclusion is reached that interpersonal difficulties are a problem to address, we suggest that it may be helpful to target a patient's interpersonal problems at the same time as addressing the eating disorder. In this case, we add "life" to the patients' personal formulation (Fig. 5.5).

5.3.3 Strategies for Addressing Marked Interpersonal Difficulties

The goals are to resolve current interpersonal difficulties (e.g. conflicts, role transitions, or difficulties in forming and maintaining relationships) and enhance interpersonal functioning (e.g. quality of relationships, appropriate assertiveness). The

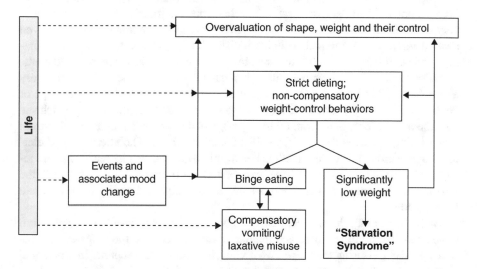

Fig. 5.5 The interaction of marked interpersonal difficulties ("LIFE") with the eating-disorder psychopathology. Reproduced with permission from the Online Training Programme in CBT-E, CREDO Oxford, 2017

strategies used to address marked interpersonal difficulties in the context of CBT-E
for eating disorders have been described in a previous publication [2], and involve
the application of the following procedures:

- Addressing social isolation and interpersonal functioning deficits

  – Providing personalized education
  – Analysing repetitive dysfunctional behaviours
  – Learning to use assertive communication
  – Addressing interpersonal avoidance
  – Developing new interests and relationships

- Addressing interpersonal conflicts

  – Providing personalized education
  – Dealing with interpersonal conflicts

- Addressing role transitions

  – Providing personalized education
  – Reviewing the positive and negative aspects of the old and new roles
  – Exploring thoughts and emotions associated with role change
  – Developing new social skills
  – Developing new interests and relationships

Vignette

The patient is a 19-year-old female whose problems with eating began at age 18, a
few months after she had begun studying Medicine at university in another city. In
high school she had been the best in her class, but the transition to university was
very difficult because she suffered from loneliness (it was the first time she had lived
away from home); she was also finding it difficult to study some subjects (e.g. anat-
omy and chemistry), and felt threatened by greater competition from other students.
Because she had lost touch with all of her friends from high school, she felt very
alone. She also felt out of control and, since she was dissatisfied with the shape of
her body, she severely restricted her diet. However, after 1 month, during which she
lost about 3 kg (dropping from 60 to 57 kg), her diet was interrupted by recurrent
binge-eating episodes followed by self-induced vomiting. The alternation of dieting, binge eating and vomiting halted her weight loss, and this increased her preoccupation with her weight and shape, manifested via frequent body checking in the
mirror, and worsening of her mood, social relationships and ability to concentrate
on her studies.

At the beginning, she was very engaged with CBT-E but, despite the application
of self-monitoring in real time and regular eating procedures, the binge-eating episodes persisted. During the Stage Two review, it became clear that her interpersonal
circumstances were having a major influence on her eating. When she felt lonely or
stressed about her studies, she would skip lunch (abandoning regular eating), which
would lead to a binge-eating episode followed by self-induced vomiting immediately afterward.

The patient agreed that her interpersonal difficulties (i.e. role transition) were maintaining her eating disorder and had become a major obstacle to treatment progress, and in Stage Three part of each session was dedicated to addressing role transition (becoming a successful university student) as a major interpersonal problem. The therapist helped the patient to identify the hurdles that the transition would involve, but also the potential advantages. The treatment focus was on helping her to accept not being at the top of her class, but also stimulating her to actively engage in developing new friendships. At each session she reflected on what had happened during the previous week and what could be learned from it. She gradually made progress, developing a close friendship with two other students, adopting regular eating and flexible meal planning, and reducing dysfunctional body checking. At the end of the treatment, she retained some residual eating disorder features (i.e. avoidance of some foods and sporadic binge-eating episodes), but these had resolved completely by the post-treatment review session.

5.4   Mood Intolerance

In a subgroup of patients with eating disorders, eating is markedly influenced by events and associated mood changes [12]. These patients suffer from a problem called "mood intolerance" [1], which, since it maintains the eating disorder and interferes with treatment, should be directly addressed.

5.4.1   Characteristics of Mood Intolerance

Mood intolerance has two principal components [1, 13]:

1. Extreme sensitivity to intense (especially aversive) mood states characterized by an inability to accept and deal appropriately with them;
2. The use of dysfunctional mood-modulation behaviours to reduce awareness of an intense mood state and neutralize it, which comes at a personal cost.

Dysfunctional mood-modulation behaviours may be expressed via two major abnormal behaviours in people with eating disorders: (i) self-harming (e.g. cutting or burning the skin), and/or (ii) taking a psychoactive substance (e.g. alcohol, other substances). In addition, people with an eating disorder and mood intolerance often discover that certain eating disorder behaviours may be used to cope with their emotions. In this way, the binge eating, self-induced vomiting and excessive exercising can become means of modulating emotions (Fig. 5.6). In these cases, mood intolerance needs to be addressed as it is an additional mechanism maintaining the eating disorder psychopathology.

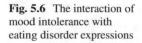

Fig. 5.6 The interaction of mood intolerance with eating disorder expressions

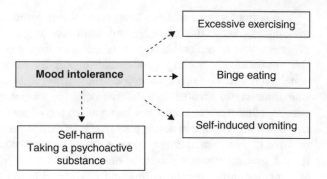

5.4.2   Assessing for the Presence of Mood Intolerance

Mood intolerance should be suspected if the patient reports a recurrent association between mood changes and some behavioural expressions of the eating disorder psychopathology, and when proactive problem-solving does not help to address this link. In any event, it is advisable to directly address mood intolerance in the following cases:

- Current or previous reports of other dysfunctional mood-modulation behaviours (e.g. self-harm or substance misuse)
- Presence of intense emotional states that stimulate and maintain certain behavioural expressions of the eating disorder psychopathology (e.g. binge eating, self-induced vomiting, excessive exercising)

5.4.3   Strategies for Addressing Mood Intolerance

The strategies used to address marked interpersonal difficulties in the context of CBT-E for eating disorders have been described in a previous publication [2, 14], and involve the application of the following procedures:

- *Education on mood intolerance.* Patients are educated on the role of mood intolerance in maintaining their eating disorder. It is underlined that some mood-modulation behaviours are dysfunctional because although they may help a person to tolerate mood changes in the short-term, they prevent the acquisition of skills for coping with intense moods in the long term and ultimately lead to impairment.
- *Analysing a recent example of mood intolerance.* The therapist reviews a recent episode of mood intolerance with the patient to re-create the sequence of seven events:
  - The occurrence of a triggering event (e.g. an argument with a friend)
  - Cognitive appraisal of the event (e.g. "She was mean to me")

- An aversive mood change (e.g. anger)
- Cognitive appraisal of the mood change, followed by rapid cognitive amplification of the mood (e.g. "I can't stand feeling angry like this"), leading to
  greater mood amplification over a short period resulting in thoughts (e.g. "I
  really can't stand feeling like this")
- The use of dysfunctional mood-modulation behaviour (e.g. binge eating or
  self-harm)
- The immediate amelioration of the aversive mood (e.g. dissipation of feeling
  of anger)
- Later cognitive appraisal (e.g. "I have no control over my eating").

- *Discussing the mechanisms involved in mood intolerance*
- *Slowing down, observing, and analysing*
- *Intervening in the sequence of events*

  - Preventing the occurrence of triggering events
  - Addressing the cognitive appraisal of events
  - Addressing aversive moods and their cognitive appraisal ("mood acceptance")
  - Introducing functional mood modulation (e.g. mood-altering music or mov-
    ies, talking to others, exercising, taking a cold shower)
  - Putting barriers in the way of dysfunctional mood modulation
  - Adopting a healthy lifestyle and making radical life changes

Vignette
The patient is a 23-year-old underweight woman, living with her mother, who
reported 3–4 episodes of self-induced vomiting daily after normal meals, and recurrent episodes of self-harm (i.e. razor cuts on the forearms). Her self-injurious behaviours had begun at the age of 18, immediately after she had been sexually assaulted
by a non-relative. After a few months, she also started to have recurrent subjective
binge-eating episodes followed by self-induced vomiting to lose weight. This
resulted in a weight loss of about 13 kg (from 54 to 48 kg) in a few months, and an
interruption in her menstrual cycle. In the following years, the patient was unsuccessfully treated via two psychological treatments that focused on the abuse, as well
as several psychopharmacological agents.

The patient, referred to us by her general practitioner, appreciated the collaborative nature of CBT-E, and immediately became engaged in the treatment. During
CBT-E Step One, with the regular eating procedure the frequency of subjective
binge-eating episodes was markedly reduced from twice a day to three times a
week. In this period, she also reported only four episodes of self-harm (using a
razor)—all three after arguments with her mother.

In Step Two of CBT-E, binge-eating and self-harm analysis revealed that these
episodes were often triggered by rapid changes in her mood. The therapist realiz-
ing that the proactive problem-solving procedure was ineffective at managing her
rapid mood swings, suggested to the patient that they address mood intolerance
directly. The patient also agreed that her mother be involved in order to create a
home environment in which there was no easy access to dangerous objects (e.g.

razors or knives), and agree to stop criticizing the patient's eating behaviour. The strategies and procedures used for addressing mood intolerance, along with the mother's assistance in creating a safe, non-critical environment, enabled the patient to stop self-harming within a few weeks. The patient realized that she was able to tolerate mood changes by accepting and managing them in a more functional way (e.g. listening to music, taking a walk, or both). The combination of these procedures, associated with those addressing undereating, dietary restraint and body image, also produced a reduction in both the frequency of subjective binge-eating episodes (which fell to once every 2–3 weeks) and the normalization of body weight (she reached 52 kg), while a moderate overvaluation of shape and weight persisted.

In the post-treatment review session, after 20 weeks, the patient reported that she had experienced no episodes of self-harm and only one episode of binge-eating over the previous 4 weeks, and that she was confident that by continuing to apply the procedures learned in CBT-E she could achieve complete remission of the eating disorder.

References

1. Fairburn CG, Cooper Z, Shafran R. Cognitive behaviour therapy for eating disorders: a "transdiagnostic" theory and treatment. Behav Res Ther. 2003;41(5):509–28. https://doi.org/10.1016/s0005-7967(02)00088-8.
2. Dalle Grave R, Calugi S. Cognitive behavior therapy for adolescents with eating disorders. New York: Guilford Press; 2020.
3. Fairburn CG, Cooper Z, Shafran R, Bohn K, Hawker DM. Clinical perfectionism, core low self-esteem and interpersonal problems. In: Fairburn CG, editor. Cognitive behavior therapy and eating disorders. New York: The Guilford Press; 2008. p. 197–221.
4. Shafran R, Cooper Z, Fairburn CG. Clinical perfectionism: a cognitive-behavioural analysis. Behav Res Ther. 2002;40(7):773–91. https://doi.org/10.1016/s0005-7967(01)00059-6.
5. Egan SJ, Wade TD, Shafran R, Antony MM. Cognitive-behavioral treatment of perfectionism. New York: Guilford Press; 2004.
6. Shafran R, Egan S, Wade T. Overcoming perfectionism: a self-help guide using scientifically supported cognitive behavioural techniques. London: Little, Brown Book Group; 2010.
7. Jones R, Peveler RC, Hope RA, Fairburn CG. Changes during treatment for bulimia nervosa: a comparison of three psychological treatments. Behav Res Ther. 1993;31(5):479–85. https://doi.org/10.1016/0005-7967(93)90128-h.
8. Fairburn CG, Cooper Z, Doll HA, Welch SL. Risk factors for anorexia nervosa: three integrated case-control comparisons. Arch Gen Psychiatry. 1999;56(5):468–76. https://doi.org/10.1001/archpsyc.56.5.468.
9. Fairburn CG, Welch SL, Doll HA, Davies BA, O'Connor ME. Risk factors for bulimia nervosa. A community-based case-control study. Arch Gen Psychiatry. 1997;54(6):509–17. https://doi.org/10.1001/archpsyc.1997.01830180015003.
10. Fennell MJ. Overcoming low self-esteem: a self-help guide using cognitive behavioural techniques. 2nd ed. London: Constable & Robinson; 2016.
11. Fennell M. Overcoming low self-esteem. London: Constable & Robinson; 2009.

12. Meyer C, Waller G, Waters A. Emotional states and bulimic psychopathology. In: Hoek HW, Treasure JL, Katzman MA, editors. Neurobiology in the treatment of eating disorders. Chichester: Wiley; 1998. p. 271–87.
13. Linehan MM. Cognitive-behavioral treatment of borderline personality disorder. New York: Guilford Press; 1993.
14. Fairburn CG, Cooper Z, Shafran R, Bohn K, Hawker D, Murphy R, et al. Enhanced cognitive behavior therapy for eating disorders: The core protocol. In: Fairburn CG, editor. Cognitive behavior therapy and eating disorders. New York: Guilford Press; 2008. p. 45–193.

Chapter 6
Coexisting Mental Disorders

As described in Chap. 4, most patients with eating disorders meet the diagnostic criteria for at least one other psychiatric disorder. The most frequently coexisting disorders are clinical depression, anxiety disorders and substance use disorders. However, most studies assessing the frequency of psychiatric comorbidities in eating disorders have had a cross-sectional or case-controlled design, and reported associations might be due to reverse causation [1]. In fact, the comorbid features observed may be the result of undereating and being underweight (starvation symptoms) and/or the underlying eating-disorder psychopathology. One strategy for overcoming this problem would be to design and conduct longitudinal general population studies [2] to assess whether psychiatric comorbidities are present before the onset of the eating disorder. However, these studies are costly and difficult to enact and are associated with a high rate of attrition, limiting the utility of their conclusions. Furthermore, patients receiving treatment today require urgent action, and this issue must therefore be addressed without the benefit of future research findings.

In the real clinical word, the assessment of a patient's psychopathology is inevitably cross-sectional and, therefore, the risk of attributing some observed features that are in fact secondary to the eating-disorder psychopathology to a comorbid psychiatric disorder is high. However, three general questions may help decide whether it might be helpful to treat a potential coexisting mental disorder as a separate entity or not [3]:

1. *Are the features of the coexisting disorder directly attributable to the eating disorder or its consequences?* If so, the apparent comorbidity could be spurious and simply represent an effect of the eating disorder itself.
2. *Are the features of the coexisting disorder likely to interfere with the treatment of the eating disorder?* If so, they must be addressed beforehand or at the same time.
3. *Are the features of the coexisting disorder likely to resolve if the eating disorder is successfully treated?* If so, and if it is unlikely that they will not interfere with the treatment, they probably do not need to be addressed directly.

R. Dalle Grave et al., *Complex Cases and Comorbidity in Eating Disorders*, https://doi.org/10.1007/978-3-030-69341-1_6

In this chapter, we describe the strategies used to assess and treat the main psychiatric disorders coexisting with eating-disorder psychopathology.

6.1 Clinical Depression

Coexisting mood disorders have been reported in more than 40% of eating disorder cases [4]. This explains why a large subgroup of patients with eating disorder receive a diagnosis of clinical depression, also known as major depression or major depressive disorder, and are treated with antidepressant medications. However, a diagnosis of coexisting clinical depression is often inappropriate [3], because there is a substantial conceptual overlap between some features of the two disorders. It is therefore not easy to discern whether the coexistence of eating disorder and depression constitutes true or spurious comorbidity, but an attempt must be made in patients seeking eating-disorder treatment in order to prevent the superfluous prescription of antidepressants.

It is well known that in anorexia nervosa many features used for the diagnosis of clinical depression are the consequences of being underweight [5]. Examples are as follows:

- Low mood
- Social withdrawal
- Heightened obsessionality and indecision
- Disturbed sleep with early waking
- Decreased energy and drive
- Loss of sexual desire
- Impaired concentration
- Irritability

Similarly, in bulimia nervosa, many features used for the diagnosis of clinical depression are known to be the consequence of recurrent binge-eating episodes [3]. Examples are as follows:

- Self-criticism
- Low mood
- Social withdrawal
- Shame
- Guilt
- Feelings of impotence

On the other side of the coin, features suggestive that there is in fact clinical depression coexisting with the eating disorder are the following [3]:

- A personal history of clinical depression before the onset of the eating disorder
- Late eating disorder onset

- Recent intensification of depressive features in the absence of any change in the eating-disorder psychopathology (e.g., low mood, social withdrawal, or suicidal thoughts and plans).
- Loss of interest, crying, recurrent thoughts on the pointlessness of life, personal neglect.

The more of these features that are reported by the patient, the more confident we are that a diagnosis of clinical depression is warranted.

The distinction between depression secondary to the eating disorder and coexisting clinical depression is essential for an optimal therapeutic intervention. In the former case, the depressive features should not be treated because they tend to resolve alongside an improvement in the eating-disorder psychopathology. Indeed, addressing the consequences of eating disorder with a pharmacological or psychological treatment designed for another psychiatric disorder may increase the risk of deviating from the treatment of the eating-disorder psychopathology and, in any case, expose the patients to side effects without the possibility of achieving significant improvements.

In contrast, coexisting clinical depression must be identified and treated because it hinders the treatment of the eating disorder itself. Those suffering from coexisting clinical depression think that it is not possible to change, have little energy to engage in treatment, and too poor concentration to understand and retain the information provided. In these cases, we recommend a pharmacological treatment (antidepressants) for 9–12 months, after having educated the patients and obtained their informed consent. The decision to use antidepressants rather than a psychological treatment to address the coexisting clinical depression is based on two principal observations [3]: (i) psychological treatment of clinical depression requires a lot of time, and progress is limited by the presence of the eating disorder as the two psychopathologies negatively interact; and (ii) antidepressants, in particular SSRIs (e.g., fluoxetine and sertraline), generally work rapidly and well.

If a patient has reservations about taking antidepressants, they should be informed that these psychopharmacologial agents do not interfere with the ability to do things in life, and that the resolution of clinical depression will allow them to be in the best condition to handle psychological treatment of their eating disorder. In addition, antidepressant drugs are not addictive, they are not mood enhancers (they only treat depression), and have few side effects (e.g., nausea), which are usually transient and last only a few days. The patient should be reassured that should they develop more persistent side effects, such as a fine hand tremor, difficulty swallowing, and decrease or loss of sexual desire, their antidepressant regime will be reassessed. Eating disorder patients will also be interested to know that SSRIs do not increase appetite although fluoxetine at higher doses (60 mg daily) can reduce the propensity to binge eat. They should be warned that SSRIs are, however, associated with a greater sensitivity to the intoxicating effects of alcohol, and so be advised to drink with caution.

Patients with severe clinical depression refusing antidepressants may nevertheless be offered an inpatient CBT-E-based treatment that targets both coexisting disorders simultaneously. Indeed, a study conducted by our team found no significant differences in the outcomes of inpatient CBT-E between eating-disorder patients with or without clinical depression [6]. Table 6.1 shows a summary of the

Table 6.1 CBT-E recommendations for assessing and treating coexisting clinical depression in eating disorders

Clinical features that suggest the presence of coexisting clinical depression
• Recent intensification of depressive features (in the absence of changes in eating-disorder psychopathology)
• Pervasive and extreme negative thoughts (beyond the concerns about shape, weight, eating and their control)
– Global negative thoughts
– A general sense of helplessness (e.g., seeing the future as bleak, resignation)
– Recurring thoughts of death
– Thoughts and plans for suicide
– Guilt regarding events and circumstances not related to the eating disorder
• A decrease in interest and involvement with others (in addition to any impairment previously caused by the eating disorder)
– Decrease in socialization
– Disruption of usual activities (e.g., reading the newspaper, listening to the radio, reading the mail, paying bills)
• A decrease in energy and the ability to make decisions
– A decrease in the ability to motivate oneself to do the usual things (e.g., working, playing sports)
– Procrastination
• Other features
– Frequent crying
– Failure to maintain personal hygiene and physical appearance
– Late onset of eating disorder (e.g., after 30 years of age)
– Atypical moods within the sessions (e.g., persistent low mood, frequent crying)
– Poor response to the first phase of treatment
– Failure to do homework between sessions due to lack of interest and energy
Treatment of coexisting clinical depression
• Fluoxetine
– Prescribe 40 mg to be taken in the morning before eating (patients with eating disorders do not usually respond to lower doses)
– After 2 weeks, re-evaluate the patient (results are usually evident after 10–12 days); if the response is positive continue with 40 mg, otherwise increase to 60 mg daily and wait for another 2–3 weeks. If patients do not have a sufficient response, increase to 80 mg (some patients may reach 100 mg daily)
– Continue therapy with fluoxetine for 9 months to minimize the risk of relapse
– Monitor side effects
Transient side effects such as nausea may appear in the first 5 days and then disappear
Persistent side effects such as fine hand tremor, difficulty swallowing or a reduced or loss of libido should prompt reassessment and likely a change in antidepressant

strategies used for assessing and treating coexisting clinical depression in eating disorders according to CBT-E recommendations [3, 7].

Vignette

The patient is a 28-year-old woman with severe and enduring anorexia nervosa (see Chap. 9). The patient reported the onset of the eating disorder at the age of 14, with the adoption of a strict low-calorie diet to lose weight and to change the shape of her legs. The course of the eating disorder was characterized by the persistent maintenance of severe and extreme dietary restriction and progressive weight loss, and the onset of secondary amenorrhea.

The patient had had numerous specialized outpatient treatments and been hospitalized without ever obtaining any improvements in her eating-disorder psychopathology or body weight, which has remained stable at around 35–37 kg. In the last year, the patient has been consulting a general psychiatrist who, due to the presence of depressed mood, social isolation and loss of sexual desire, diagnosed a major depressive disorder and prescribed fluoxetine, subsequently enhanced with a combination of olanzapine and sodium valproate. However, drug treatment did not result in any improvement in the eating-disorder psychopathology or depression, and the patient's general practitioner referred her to us for possible hospitalization in a specialist eating disorder unit.

At the assessment and preparation session, the patient weighted 35 kg (BMI 13.5), and reported following extreme and rigid dietary rules over the last 28 days, with a caloric intake not to exceed 800 kcal per day. She also reported intense fear of gaining weight; overvaluation of shape, weight, eating and their control; low mood; asthenia; social withdrawal and decreased sexual desire. The patient was initially very ambivalent about the proposal of being hospitalized, but after four preparatory sessions with a CBT-E psychologist from our team decided to be admitted and to play an active role in the treatment.

Considering the absence of beneficial effects of psychopharmacological treatment and the absence of clinical features that suggested the presence of coexisting clinical depression (Table 5.1), during the initial weeks of hospitalization the team's psychiatrist received the patient's informed consent to gradually reduce and then suspend all medication. After only 4 weeks of nutritional rehabilitation and 4 kg weight regain, the patient showed a marked improvement in mood tone, asthenia and socialization, which further improved as treatment progressed. At discharge, after 20 weeks (13 in hospital and 7 in day hospital) the patient had achieved a body weight of 55 kg (BMI 19.1) and had stable mood tone, despite retaining moderate residual dietary restraint and concern about her body shape.

Vignette

The patient is a 19-year-old woman. Her eating disorder onset was at the age of 14 years, with the adoption of dietary restriction, which resulted in progressive weight loss from 56 kg up to 46 kg, and secondary amenorrhea. After about

1 year, the dietary restriction was interrupted by the onset of recurrent binge-eating episodes followed by self-induced vomiting, and her body weight increased to 68 kg.

She was given a generic psychological treatment for about 2 years without obtaining any improvement in her eating-disorder psychopathology. However, after the interruption of the psychological treatment, the patients reported a reduction in the frequency of her binge-eating episodes and mitigation of dietary restriction. This resulted in a gradual reduction of body weight until she reached 55 kg, a weight that she maintained for about one and a half years, despite sporadic binge-eating episodes followed by self-induced vomiting.

At the assessment and preparation session, the patient reported that over the previous 6 months, in association with the separation of her parents, she had experienced an increase in her concerns about her control of eating, weight and, to a lesser extent, body shape. These concerns led her to adopt extreme and rigid dietary rules and excessive exercising, resulting in a progressive weight loss to her current body weight of 50 kg (BMI 19.2).

During the interview, the patient had frequent episodes of crying, which were accentuated when the therapist asked about the separation of her parents and the effects that this event had had on her life. The patient also reported persistent low mood, difficulties in concentration, loss of interest, devaluing and negative thoughts about herself characterized by continuing doubts about being able to complete her studies, and accentuation of intolerance to unforeseen events.

The therapist informed the patient of the possible coexistence and interaction of clinical depression and eating disorder, and the need for treatment with antidepressants before outpatient CBT-E could be started. However, the patient preferred not to take the medicine as she was against the use of psychopharmacological treatments, and wished to begin the psychological treatment directly.

However, during CBT-E Stage One, the patient reported difficulties in performing real-time self-monitoring and applying the regular eating procedure because she considered everything she was doing to be pointless. Addressing these difficulties in the session, it emerged how clinical depression was interacting with her eating-disorder psychopathology and preventing the patient from benefiting from the CBT-E strategies and procedures. The patient agreed to consult the team psychiatrist, who prescribed her 40 mg fluoxetine per day, raised to 60 mg after a week. After about 2 weeks of drug treatment, the patient reported a marked improvement in mood tone, which was expressed in her greater and willingness to fill in her monitoring records in real time and to play an active role in the application of the regular eating procedure.

At the end of the 20 sessions of CBT-E, the patient had achieved a body weight of 52 kg, and reported stable mood and a reduction in dietary restraint and concerns about weight and eating control. The treatment with fluoxetine continued for about a year and then, as per the psychiatrist's advice, was discontinued.

6.1.1 Other Mood Disorders

Sometimes we see patients with eating disorder and comorbid bipolar I or bipolar II disorder. In these cases, as long as their mood is euthymic, CBT-E can proceed without obstacles, and patients often achieve remission of their eating-disorder psychopathology. Any setbacks, which in these patients are often stimulated by changes of mood, can be effectively addressed through CBT-E strategies and procedures [3].

The management of patients with eating disorder and comorbid bipolar disorder with rapid alternation of depressive and manic or hypomanic states over a matter of days is, however, more complex. Their rapid mood changes represent an obstacle to CBT-E, and it is advisable that such patients' mood be stabilized before psychological treatment is begun [3]. Unfortunately, most pharmacological mood stabilizers (lithium carbonate, carbamazepine, gabapentin, pregabalin, sodium valproate, oxcarbazepine, etc.) negatively affect eating control, and are associated with weight gain: two side effects that may be unacceptable to some patients with eating disorders.

6.2 Anxiety Disorders

Anxiety disorders are the most frequent coexisting psychiatric comorbidity in eating disorders, and have been reported in more than 50% of cases [4]. The available data also suggest that anxiety disorders often precede the onset of eating disorders [8–10], and this has led to the speculation that they may in fact predispose affected people to develop an eating disorder. Although the prevalence of eating disorders has been observed to be high in patients who seek treatment for anxiety disorders, the research conducted in this field to date is still minimal [11]. Furthermore, the data produced has not been consistent, which complicates our understanding of the nature of the coexistence of eating disorders with anxiety disorders [11].

Although common, a comorbid anxiety disorder does not generally pose major problems for the management of an eating disorder in the way that clinical depression does. If, however, the patient presents symptoms of both anxiety disorder and clinical depression, it is possible that the anxiety is secondary to the depression; if this is indeed the case, it further grounds for the recommendation that clinical depression be treated directly, as per the indications described in the Sect. 6.1.

As with depressive features, it is also possible that the anxious state arises from the eating disorder. Hence, when a patient with an eating disorder shows some features of anxiety, the first question to ask is [3] as follows: *"Are the anxiety features directly attributable to the eating disorder or its consequences?"* An example of anxiety features secondary to the eating disorder is avoiding to socialize due to difficulties in eating in front of others or exposing body shape. These features are not indicative of social phobia because the excessive anxiety and fear are directly attributable to the eating-disorder psychopathology.

The second question to ask is [3] as follows: "*Are the anxiety features likely to interfere with the treatment of the eating disorder?*" If the comorbid anxiety disorder is real and not spurious, this is likely to occur. For example, a person with extreme agoraphobia may have difficulty attending the sessions. In this event, the agoraphobia should be treated first and then the eating disorder.

The third question to ask is as follows: "*Are the anxiety features likely to resolve if the eating disorder is successfully treated?*". In our clinical experience, this happens frequently, even when a patient has generalized anxiety disorder or social phobia with marked fear or anxiety about social situations unrelated to eating or body exposure. In these cases, if the anxiety disorder does not hinder treatment, we do not seek to treat it directly, but instead proceed with CBT-E alone. Table 6.2 describes the principal features of anxiety disorders.

Vignette

The patient is a 15-year-old teenager who suffers from anorexia nervosa and social anxiety disorder. The patient reported that she had been a shy child from infancy, but that the striking symptoms of social phobia only began to manifest during her first year of secondary school, when she began to experience fear and anxiety in various social situations that could leave her exposed to potential judgment by others (e.g., oral examinations at school, speaking with unknown people); in such situations she feared that she would be judged poorly, humiliated and rejected. As a result, she began to avoid many social situations or, when she had no choice but to undertake them (e.g., an oral exam at school), the exposure was associated with intense fear and anxiety, which she often handled by eating sweets and junk food between meals.

This behaviour was associated with progressive weight gain, and at the age of 14, in the summer preceding the beginning of the first year of high school, her body weight had reached 65 kg. She began a strict diet and started exercising excessively

Table 6.2 Clinical features of anxiety disorders

Anxiety disorders include disorders that share features of excessive fear, anxiety and related behavioural disturbances [12]. Fear is the emotional response to a perceived imminent threat, while anxiety is the anticipation of future threat. These two emotional states appear very similar, but differ in some features. Fear is more often associated with surges of autonomic arousal to fight or flight, thoughts of imminent danger and escape behaviours. In contrast, anxiety is more frequently associated with muscle tension and alertness in preparation for future harm, and prudent or avoidant behaviours. Sometimes the levels of fear or anxiety are reduced by pervasive avoidance behaviours. Panic attacks, although not limited to anxiety disorders, are a particular type of fear response.

Anxiety disorders differ from normative or transient fear and anxiety because they are excessive and persistent, usually lasting longer than 6 months. Anxiety disorders also differ from each other in the type of objects or situations that induce fear, anxiety or behavioural avoidance and associated cognitive processes. Many anxiety disorders develop in childhood and tend to persist if they are not treated. They affect females more frequently than males (ratio 2:1) and should not be diagnosed when symptoms are attributable to the effects of a substance or drug or other medical condition, or are better explained by another mental disorder. For this reason, when **fear and/or anxiety and avoidance behaviours are related to eating, shape and weight, the diagnosis of an eating disorder, not of anxiety disorder, should be made.**

to lose weight, so as to be in shape when she started her new school. Such behaviours resulted in progressive weight loss, and she ended up weighing 57 kg. However, her periods stopped, and the weight loss was associated with an intensification in her social anxiety, which led to her avoiding social relationships and feeling unable to go to school.

Under pressure from her parents, she had seen a psychologist for 3 months; the main focus of the intervention was management of her social phobia, but with no appreciable success. At the CBT-E assessment and preparation session, the patient had a body weight of 47 kg (BMI 16.0) and reported following extreme and rigid dietary rules (she would not eat more than 1000 kcal per day); excessive exercising (she almost always stood and walked for many hours each day), intense fear of gaining weight; overvaluation of shape, weight, eating and their control; and frequent and dysfunctional body checking (she weighed herself several times a day and spent a lot of time looking her body in the mirror), in addition to anxiety and fear when exposed to the judgment of others, social withdrawal and interrupted school attendance.

After being educated about her eating problem and the collaborative nature of CBT-E, the patient decided that she would start outpatient treatment. As agreed to by the patient and her parents, the treatment was solely focused on addressing the eating-disorder psychopathology, not her social phobia. After the 4 weeks of CBT-E Step One, the patient decided to address weight regain, and in about 25 weeks reached a BMI-for-age percentile corresponding to a BMI of 20 in adults (59 kg). The normalization of her weight was associated with the return of a regular menstrual cycle, and marked reduction in her previous concerns about shape and weight, and her fear of gaining weight lessened considerably. However, she still found it extremely difficult to address social eating and body avoidance due to interference from her comorbid social phobia. For this reason, the therapist, in agreement with the patient, decided to use the marked interpersonal difficulties module of broad CBT-E, which is designed to help such patients to effectively cope with the difficulties related to fear of the judgment of others. The treatment was associated with remission of the eating-disorder psychopathology and a marked reduction of fear and anxiety in social situations. This permitted the patient to resume attending school and establish friendships.

6.2.1 Eating-Disorder Psychopathology Is Not a Specific Form of Phobia

The psychological conceptualization of anorexia nervosa has been dominated for many years by the avoidance paradigm, according to which the probability of a behaviour increases if it is followed by negative reinforcement (i.e., removal of the aversive stimulus). If applied to anorexia nervosa, this model explains most of the distinctive behavioural expressions of the disorder (e.g., strict dieting, excessive exercising, self-induced vomiting, and laxative and diuretics misuse), which are adopted for the purpose of avoiding specific aversive stimuli, i.e., weight gain and getting fat [13].

The avoidance model is also compatible with the conceptualization of anorexia nervosa as an adaptive disorder in which "weight phobia" represents the avoidance of the feared circumstances associated with psychosexual maturity [14]. According to this theory, weight loss becomes a means of avoiding the challenges associated with psychosexual development, for which the person with anorexia nervosa feels unprepared. Although in most cases the source of this phobia (the aversive stimulus) is not expressed by patients, some authors have reported that it is often associated with issues concerning sexuality, high performance standards, separation from family or family conflicts [13].

This avoidance model postulates that the avoidance, once acquired, is maintained by the persistent eating-disorder behaviours, which isolate the individual from the possibility of recognizing when the aversive contingencies are no longer operating. Cognitive variables seem to contribute in part to this process as the avoidance prevents the development of inhibitory learning of fear by not allowing falsification of the occurrence of the feared consequences [15, 16].

However, the conceptualization of anorexia nervosa as a phobic disorder is difficult to maintain because the control of shape and weight seen in this disorder is often associated with a sense of triumph, mastery, self-control and superiority in its sufferers [13]. It is common to observe this feature in the accounts of patients who, especially in the early phases of their weight loss, report being "happy", "exultant", "satisfied", "powerful" and "proud". Indeed, weight loss is often experienced as a "goal", "an achievement", "a virtue", "a source of positive pleasure" and/or "a sensual pleasure" [17].

This sets eating-disorder psychopathology apart from a simple "weight phobia"; indeed, people with agoraphobia experience a severe state of anxiety when they are in open spaces, but generally do not report a feeling of euphoria or a sense of power when they are indoors [18]. Furthermore, individuals with agoraphobia tend to perceive their anxiety as excessive and uncontrollable, and use the strategy of avoidance to eliminate this anxiety. Those with anorexia nervosa, on the other hand, often perceive their preoccupation with shape, weight, eating and their control, and the associated negative mood states (e.g., anxiety), as useful means of keeping control over their shape and weight [19].

The egosyntonic characteristics of anorexia nervosa have led the positive cognitive reinforcement associated with the control of shape and weight to be considered as the core psychopathology of this eating disorder [19, 20]. Indeed, according to the modern transdiagnostic cognitive behavioural theory, as described in Chap. 3 (Sect. 3.2), a distinctive self-evaluation scheme, the overvaluation of shape, weight and their control (i.e., judging oneself predominantly or exclusively in terms of shape, weight and their control), is of central importance in maintaining anorexia nervosa, and also other eating disorders [21]. According to this theory, most other clinical features of this eating disorder, including weight phobia, derive from this specific core psychopathology.

Identification of the core psychopathology of anorexia nervosa is important not only for academic purposes; above all, it has significant implications for the psychological treatment of this disorder. Indeed, evidence-based CBT-E [7, 21], derived from the transdiagnostic theory, differs considerably from behavioural exposure-based programmes as it is not designed to primarily address weight phobia. On the contrary, CBT-E seeks to actively involve patients in the implementation of strategies and procedures that make feel them in control when addressing the main expressions and maintenance factors of the disorder, with the ultimate aim of their developing a more articulated and functional self-evaluation scheme, one that is less dependent on their shape, weight and eating control.

6.3   Obsessive-Compulsive Disorder

The coexistence of eating disorders with obsessive-compulsive disorder reportedly ranges from 10 to 40% in patients with anorexia nervosa, and affects up to 40% of patients with bulimia nervosa [22, 23]. Furthermore, among patients who received a primary diagnosis of obsessive-compulsive disorder, a coexisting eating disorder has been observed in about 11% of cases [24]. However, in a large subgroup of patients with eating disorder, the diagnosis of obsessive-compulsive disorder is often made in response to typical features of the eating-disorder such as "obsessive and compulsive" adherence to eating rituals and/or excessive exercising, and is therefore misplaced.

Indeed, eating rituals are common in patients with anorexia nervosa and are often accentuated by caloric restriction and being underweight. In fact, these behaviours were even reported in the Minnesota Starvation Experiment participants (see Chap. 2, Sect. 2.2), who underwent a prolonged period of semistarvation without having any features of eating-disorder psychopathology [5]. Only later were these features recognized as "starvation symptoms" by clinicians, when they noted their presence in patients with anorexia nervosa. The most frequent eating rituals observed are stirring food, separating the food to be eaten, counting bites, cutting food into geometric shapes, cutting food into small pieces, chewing for a long time, taking long breaks between bites and eating extremely slowly.

Excessive exercising is also a common feature of patients with eating disorders, particularly those of low weight. In a sample of patients admitted to Villa Garda Hospital, for example, excessive exercising was observed in 45.5% of cases, with the highest prevalence (80%) in those diagnosed with restrictive anorexia nervosa [25]. Excessive exercising has two distinctive characteristics [26]: (i) its duration, frequency and intensity exceeds what is necessary to obtain health benefits, and increases the risk of producing physical damage; and (ii) it is associated with a subjective sense of being forced or compelled, taking priority over other day-to-day activities and causing guilt or anxiety if postponed.

Therefore, in CBT-E eating rituals and excessive exercising are considered a direct expression of the core psychopathology of eating disorders (i.e., the overvaluation of shape, weight, eating and their control), and are mainly used to manage concerns about shape, weight and eating control (Fig. 6.1). However, some clinicians tend to confuse these two specific features of the eating-disorder psychopathology as features of an obsessive-compulsive disorder, given the rigidity and persistence with which they are applied. To prevent misunderstanding, the DSM-5 clearly states, in criterion D of the obsessive-compulsive disorder diagnosis, that the disorder should not be explained by the symptoms of other mental disorders, among which it includes the ritualized eating behaviours of eating disorders [12]. In addition, in the "differential diagnosis" section the DSM-5 specifies that obsessive-compulsive disorder can be distinguished from anorexia nervosa because in the former obsessions and compulsions are not limited to concerns about shape and weight.

Another element that distinguishes the two psychopathologies is the egosyntonic nature of the patients' concerns. Specifically, patients with eating disorder perceive preoccupation with food and eating as functional to the control of weight and body shape. In contrast, those with obsessive-compulsive disorder judge the obsessions as intrusive and harmful.

The above considerations underline the importance of assessing psychopathology to achieve an accurate diagnosis of mental disorders, and how merely relying on observation of symptoms is frequently flawed and misleading. Furthermore, a

Fig. 6.1 A formulation showing that eating rituals and excessive exercising are the expression of the overvaluation of shape, weight, eating, and their control

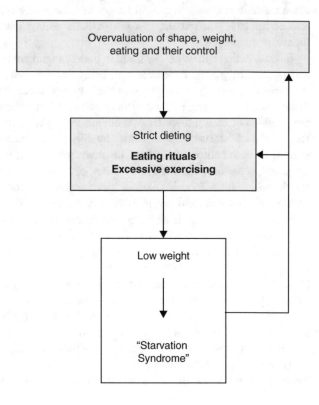

misdiagnosis of obsessive-compulsive disorder exposes patients to inadequate psychological and psychopharmacological treatments that can aggravate and maintain eating disorder psychopathology.

When obsessive-compulsive disorder does coexist with an eating disorder, and the patient's obsessions and compulsions are not solely focused on concerns about food and eating, the question arises as to when to address the two disorders. Obsessive-compulsive disorder does not generally interfere with the treatment of eating disorders but does not respond to it either. It must therefore be recognized and a decision made on when to address it with psychological treatment. This should be before or after, but preferably not at the same time. In most cases, we opt to address the eating-disorder psychopathology first because, as seen in the Minnesota Starvation Experiment (see Chap. 2, Sect. 2.2), being underweight accentuates the frequency and intensity of obsessions. We also often combine a psychopharmacological treatment for obsessive-compulsive disorder with CBT-E, although in underweight and undereating patients its effect may be limited.

Much more problematic, though rare, are cases of obsessive-compulsive disorder in which obsessions and compulsions influence the patient's eating and, therefore, act to maintain the eating-disorder psychopathology. In such cases patients tend to report that eating rituals are used to manage some obsessions not related to the control of shape and weight (e.g., "If I do not cut food into geometric shapes, something bad will happen"; "If I eat the last bite, this moment will disappear forever and I will never get it back"; "Something irreparable could happen if I eat quickly"; "If I eat some foods, I will be contaminated"). In these cases, the obsessive-compulsive disorder should be addressed first, or the two disorders can be treated at the same time by the same therapist, although this option is complex and requires skills that few therapists possess. Table 6.3 describes the principal features of obsessive-compulsive disorder.

Vignette
The patient is a 14-year-old only child suffering from anorexia nervosa and obsessive-compulsive disorder. She was referred to us by her family doctor after showing no improvement in family-based therapy, mainly focused on "dysfunctional" relationships between family members.

Her obsessions, which arose in childhood, concerned fear of contamination by germs, bacteria or viruses that could be found in "contaminated" substances, such as objects, people's skin and sweat, urine and faeces. To avoid any possibility of contamination, the patient adopted specific compulsions, including prolonged handwashing, cleaning the bathroom and objects for a long time, and refusing to touch objects or people's hands.

At the age of 13 and a body weight of 58 kg (BMI 23.0), after having been teased about the shape of her rear by her classmates, she embarked upon a low-calorie diet to lose weight and change the shape of her body. This resulted in progressive weight loss and the onset of secondary amenorrhea. Her weight loss was associated with an intensification of her obsessions and compulsions about contamination and, as a

Table 6.3 Clinical features of obsessive-compulsive disorder

Obsessive-compulsive disorder is characterized by the presence of obsessions and/or compulsions [12].
Obsessions are recurrent and persistent thoughts, urges or images experienced as intrusive and unwanted, which, in most people, cause marked anxiety or discomfort. The subject attempts to ignore or suppress such thoughts, impulses or images, or to neutralize them with other thoughts or actions (i.e., by implementing a compulsive behaviour).
Compulsions are repetitive behaviours (e.g., washing hands, tidying up, controlling) or mental actions (e.g., praying, counting, repeating words mentally) that the subject feels obliged to implement in response to the obsession, or according to rules that must be applied rigidly. Such behaviours or actions are aimed at preventing or reducing anxiety or discomfort, or preventing certain dreaded events or situations. However, these behaviours or mental actions are not realistically linked with what they are designed to neutralize or prevent, or are excessive.
Obsessions or compulsions are time-consuming (taking up more than an hour a day) or cause clinically significant discomfort or impairment of functioning in social, work or other important spheres.
Obsessive-compulsive disorder should be diagnosed only when symptoms are not attributable to the effects of a substance or drug or other medical condition, or not better explained by another mental disorder. For this **reason, when the ritualized eating behaviour or obsessions and compulsions are limited to concerns about shape and weight, obsessive-compulsive disorder should not be diagnosed.**

consequence, the patient spent hours washing her hands and taking long showers to get rid of the feeling of dirtiness, and reduce the risk of being infected with germs.

In the 3 months before being referred to our unit, the patient reported a weight loss of about 5 kg, following extreme and rigid dietary rules (she ate mainly fruits and vegetables and some rice cakes), excessive exercising (walking for many hours during the day), intense fear of weight gain, marked concerns about shape and weight, and frequent body checking in mirrors. In addition, she reported frequent mood swings, irritability, intense obsessions, and contamination compulsions that occupied many hours each day, as well as social withdrawal and interruption of school attendance. Medical examination showed marked protein malnutrition, a BMI of 13.8, and dermatitis of the hands, with dry skin, micro-cuts and slight abrasions from excessive washing. Given the severity of malnutrition and her eating-disorder psychopathology and obsessive-compulsive disorder, the assessing physician recommended inpatient CBT-E. The patient was initially ambivalent, but after four preparation sessions accepted hospitalization and agreed to play an active role in the treatment to address weight regain and the eating-disorder psychopathology.

Upon her arrival in the unit, the team decided that due to the marked malnutrition, weight loss and accentuation of obsessive and compulsive symptoms, to focus the psychological intervention solely on the eating-disorder psychopathology and weight restoration, and to treat the obsessive-compulsive disorder with sertraline. The patient and parents agreed, and in fact the patient immediately became engaged in the treatment, developing a good therapeutic relationship and actively participating in the various phases of inpatient CBT-E by applying the agreed therapeutic strategies. At the end of the inpatient treatment, the obsessive-compulsive psychopathology was in remission, and the eating-disorder psychopathology had significantly improved. The patient reported only moderate levels of dietary restraint, with some residual rigid dietary rules and concerns about body shape, which were successfully addressed in the 20 weeks of post-inpatient CBT-E.

6.4 Post-Traumatic Stress Disorder

Exposure to trauma, particularly sexual abuse in childhood, is considered a non-specific risk factor for the onset of eating disorders [27]. Although it is not known how the mechanism by which trauma contributes to the aetiology of eating disorders, it has been suggested that the development of post-traumatic stress disorder (PTSD) may mediate the relationship between trauma and eating disorder [28].

The National Women's Study found that 36.9% of participants with bulimia nervosa, 21% with binge-eating disorder and 11.8% of women who did not have these two disorders met the diagnostic criteria for lifetime PTSD [29]. These figures were confirmed by the National Comorbidity Survey-Replication Study, which found comorbid PTSD in 39% of participants with bulimia nervosa, 25% with binge-eating disorder and 16% with nervous anorexia [30].

The coexistence of eating disorder and PTSD has not, however, been much studied, in part because the two disorders have different clinical presentations (Table 6.4). That being said, we have encountered patients who improperly received a diagnosis of PTSD because they had a reported history of abuse and impulsive behaviour

Table 6.4 Clinical features of post-traumatic stress disorder

The essential feature of post-traumatic stress disorder (PTDS) is the development of characteristic symptoms, lasting more than 1 month, as a result of exposure to one or more traumatic events (e.g., death or threat of death, serious injury or sexual violence) experienced directly or indirectly [12]. These symptoms create clinically significant discomfort or psychosocial impairment and should not be attributable to the intake of substances or medications. The characteristic symptoms, which can have a variable presentation in different individuals, can be divided into four main categories:

1. Presence of recurrent, involuntary and intrusive symptoms related to the event (e.g., memories, dreams, flashbacks)

2. Attempts to avoid situations, people, places or anything else that may evoke the traumatic experience

3. Negative changes in thoughts and emotions (e.g., persistent negative emotional state, loss of interest in significant activities, sense of detachment from others)

4. Marked reactivity (e.g., irritability, hypervigilance, angry outbursts, difficulty concentrating, difficulty sleeping)

In some individuals, fear-based re-experiencing (emotional and behavioural) may be prevalent, while in others the most obvious and disturbing clinical features may relate to the loss of interest in activities previously considered pleasant (anhedonia) and low mood (dysphoria). In some individuals, arousal and reactive-externalizing symptoms are prominent, while in others altered states of consciousness, memory or identity (dissociation) predominate. Finally, some individuals show a combination of these symptom patterns.

(self-harm), in whom thorough exploration of their history revealed the presence of eating disorder features before the onset of trauma. We have also seen patients who have been erroneously diagnosed with PTSD because their recurrent binge-eating and self-induced vomiting episodes had been considered means of their escaping the trauma-induced dissociative state.

According to CBT-E theory [21] and in our clinical experience, PTSD is a separate form of psychopathology from that of an eating disorder. It does not seem to interact with the eating disorder, and does not hinder treatment. When a patient has PTSD coexisting with the eating-disorder psychopathology, we usually discuss with them which problem to address first because it is not advisable to implement two psychological treatments at the same time. In our experience, most patients choose to address eating disorder first. In this case, we seek the patient's agreement to reassess the PTSD at the end of eating disorder treatment, and, if indicated, we suggest applicable treatment options.

We also adopt the same strategy with patients who have a reported history of sexual or physical abuse, guided by data from our study comparing short- and medium-term outcomes of inpatient CBT-E in 81 patients with anorexia nervosa with or without reported sexual abuse [31]. Assessment with a semi-structured interview revealed that 24.7% of patients (n. 20) had experienced sexual abuse before the onset of anorexia nervosa, while 75.3% (61) reported no such traumatic experiences. The two groups had similar characteristics before the onset of treatment, and achieved similar improvements in BMI, eating-disorder psychopathology, general psychopathology and work and social functioning from baseline to 12 months of follow-up. Although not conclusive, these findings appear to indicate that sexual abuse in childhood does not appear to compromise the outcome of intensive CBT-E in patients with anorexia nervosa, despite the fact that the treatment does not directly address the history of sexual abuse.

Vignette
The patient is an 18-year-old female with bulimia nervosa. The eating disorder onset occurred, with recurrent binge-eating episodes, at the age of 16 years, about a year after the patient had been sexually assaulted by a 22-year-old man she had met at a disco. The course of the eating disorder was characterized by an initial weight gain of about 10 kg (from 56 to 66 kg) followed by a rapid weight loss to her lowest weight of 50 kg, in association with the adoption of extreme and rigid dietary rules and self-induced vomiting after binge-eating episodes. The patient underwent psychological treatment focused on the trauma for 1 year without obtaining any improvement in eating-disorder psychopathology.

At our unit, the patient reported a stable body weight (57 kg, BMI 21.0), recurrent binge-eating episodes (once or twice a day) followed by self-induced vomiting, following extreme and rigid dietary rules between binge-eating episodes, recurrent episodes of self-harm (cuts to the arms with a razor blade), overvaluation of shape and weight, frequent and rapid mood swings, irritability, episodes of anger towards her parents, limited socialization, and difficulty in concentrating in the 3 months preceding assessment. The patient was living with her parents and attending the last year of high school.

In CBT-E Stage One, with the adoption of the regular eating procedure, the frequency of the patient's binge-eating episodes decreased, and, as a result, so did her concerns about eating. She also reported a reduction in her concern about her weight, likely as a result of the collaborative in-session weighing, and an increase in her motivation to overcome her eating disorder. The treatment then focused on addressing her overvaluation of shape and weight, residual dietary restraint, events and mood changes associated with the use of dysfunctional mood modulation behaviours (i.e., self-harm and binge-eating). Finally, the treatment included strategies and procedures to address setbacks and prevent relapse. The erosion of the core processes maintaining the eating-disorder psychopathology resulted in complete remission from binge-eating episodes and self-induced vomiting, as well as stabilization of mood, increased socialization, and improved ability to concentrate on her studies, without the sexual trauma being directly addressed. At the post-treatment review session, the patient's eating disorder was in remission, and she had enrolled in veterinary school.

6.5   Substance Use Disorder

Substance use disorder is the persistent use of drugs (including alcohol) despite substantial harm and adverse consequences [12]. Many eating disorder patients misuse laxatives, diuretics and slimming aids, and also misuse of other substances is not uncommon in patients with eating disorders, although in most cases it is reported by those who have recurrent binge-eating episodes [32]. Alcohol misuse is the substance use disorder that most frequently coexists with eating disorders. For example, the Swedish Twin Registry revealed the following figures for prevalence of alcohol use disorder: 22% in bulimia nervosa, 22% in anorexia nervosa binge-eating/purging type, 14% in binge-eating disorder and 12% in anorexia nervosa restricting type, in comparison to 6% in twins with no eating disorder [33]. Some eating disorder patients report frequent use of recreational drugs (e.g., marijuana or ecstasy) and a minority use of cocaine or amphetamines.

Hence, when assessing patients with eating disorder and suspected coexisting substance use disorder, it is essential to evaluate the relationship between the eating-disorder psychopathology and substance use. In some cases, the misuse of substances is a direct consequence of the eating-disorder psychopathology, with the patient using cocaine or amphetamines to control body weight, for example [3]. In other cases, mood intolerance acts to maintain both the eating-disorder psychopathology and substance use disorder. In these patients, it is common to observe an intermittent use of the substance (e.g., excessive alcohol intake in non-social settings) rather than daily use of the substance. These patients often also report other dysfunctional mood modulation behaviours such as self-harm, binge eating, self-induced vomiting and excessive exercising [3].

Second, it is important to determine whether the coexisting substance use disorder is likely to interfere with the treatment of the eating-disorder psychopathology. When the misuse of substances is continuous, and the patient is intoxicated during the day, this will inevitably be the case [3], and will necessitate the patient being referred to a clinical service specialized in the treatment of substance use disorders. We generally start CBT-E after the patient has achieved lasting remission (at least 3 months) from substance misuse. If, on the other hand, the substance is being misused intermittently, as a means of weight control or to modulate emotions, we address this problem within the context of CBT-E.

The third thing to determine is whether the features of the coexisting substance use disorder are likely to resolve with remission of the eating disorder. In our clinical experience, this positive outcome occurs in many cases when substance misuse is intermittent.

We generally do not address addiction to smoking because it is rarely an obstacle to treatment. However, in the event that smoking is used as a means of resisting eating, we discourage this behaviour, and help the patient to apply the regular eating procedure instead. Trying to quit smoking while tackling an eating disorder is often too ambitious a goal, and we therefore advise our patients to postpone the attempt until after completion of CBT-E.

Vignette

The patient is a 21-year-old woman with bulimia nervosa who has requested treatment at our clinical service. She reported the onset of eating disorder at the age of 15 years, when she weighed 58 kg (BMI 22.0), with the adoption of an extreme and rigid low-calorie diet to lose weight. The course of the eating disorder was characterized by an initial weight loss for 6 months until she reached her lowest weight, 44 kg, and secondary amenorrhoea at a weight of 48 kg. Her subsequent dieting attempts were recurrently interrupted by binge-eating episodes followed by self-induced vomiting, which produced a gradual weight regain. At the age of 19 years, the patient began to use cocaine intermittently (especially on Saturday nights), sometimes associated with alcohol misuse; she had begun to take both substances for their euphoric and appetite-suppressant effects.

The patient had unsuccessfully undergone an eclectic multidisciplinary treatment from the age of 20–21 years. This included sessions with a dietitian, a generic psychological treatment and psychopharmacological treatment with fluoxetine.

At the assessment and preparation session in our unit, the patient reported a stable body weight, recurrent binge-eating episodes in the late afternoon or at dinner time (on average once a day) followed by self-induced vomiting, adhering to extreme and rigid dietary rules (she skipped breakfast and lunch), overvaluation of shape, frequent mood swings, sleep disturbances and intermittent use of cocaine in the preceding 3 months. For about 1 year she had been involved in a romantic relationship, characterized by frequent disputes, with a fellow university student; the patient was attending law school and lived alone.

The patient was begun on CBT-E because, despite reporting recurrent episodes of cocaine use, these were intermittent, did not hinder treatment and could be addressed in CBT-E Stage Three with the strategies and procedures of the Mood Intolerance module of the broad form.

6.6   Personality Disorders

As described in Chap. 4, it is difficult to make an accurate assessment of the personality of patients with eating disorders because many observed features are actually the consequence of being underweight and/or the eating-disorder psychopathology. In addition, it is particularly problematic to make a diagnosis of personality disorder in such patients because, due to the early onset of eating disorders, most do not have a period of adult life free from the influence of the disorder. Hence, we make no attempt to diagnose personality disorder. However, we do see many patients who have previously received a diagnosis of personality disorder, and tailor their treatment accordingly by using one or two modules from broad CBT-E. Here are some examples:

- Mood Intolerance module in patients who engage in self-harm or substance misuse (often diagnosed as having borderline personality disorder)
- Clinical Perfectionism module in patients with clinical perfectionism (who often receive a diagnosis of obsessive-compulsive personality disorder)
- Core Low Self-Esteem module and/or Marked Interpersonal Difficulties module in patients with core low self-esteem (who may receive a diagnosis of avoidant or dependent personality disorder)

6.7   Other Psychiatric Disorders

More rarely, patients with eating disorders may have other mental disorders. For example, we have assessed patients with schizophrenia, conversion disorder, hypochondria, body dysmorphic disorder, and autism spectrum disorder. Again, in the attempt to understand and manage these comorbidities we ask ourselves whether their features are directly attributable to the eating disorder, whether they are likely to interfere with treatment, and whether they are likely to resolve if the eating disorder treatment is successful. This can help us decide how to proceed, but a general rule is that if a patient's other condition is stabilized, CBT-E can begin as usual, and these patients often do well; otherwise, they should be treated for the coexisting psychiatric disorder before commencing treatment for the eating disorder.

References

1. Solmi F, Bentivegna F, Bould H, Mandy W, Kothari R, Rai D, et al. Trajectories of autistic social traits in childhood and adolescence and disordered eating behaviours at age 14 years: a UK general population cohort study. J Child Psychol Psychiatry. 2020;62:75. https://doi.org/10.1111/jcpp.13255.
2. Boyd A, Golding J, Macleod J, Lawlor DA, Fraser A, Henderson J, et al. Cohort profile: the 'children of the 90s'—the index offspring of the Avon longitudinal study of parents and children. Int J Epidemiol. 2013;42(1):111–27. https://doi.org/10.1093/ije/dys064.
3. Fairburn CG, Cooper Z, Waller D. Complex cases and comorbidity. In: Fairburn CG, editor. Cognitive behavior therapy and eating disorders. New York: Guilford Press; 2008.
4. Keski-Rahkonen A, Mustelin L. Epidemiology of eating disorders in Europe: prevalence, incidence, comorbidity, course, consequences, and risk factors. Curr Opin Psychiatry. 2016;29(6):340–5. https://doi.org/10.1097/yco.0000000000000278.
5. Keys A, Brozek J, Henschel A, Mickelsen O, Taylor H. The biology of human starvation. Minneapolis: University of Minnesota Press; 1950.
6. Calugi S, El Ghoch M, Conti M, Dalle Grave R. Depression and treatment outcome in anorexia nervosa. Psychiatry Res. 2014;218(1–2):195–200. https://doi.org/10.1016/j.psychres.2014.04.024.
7. Dalle Grave R, Calugi S. Cognitive behavior therapy for adolescents with eating disorders. New York: Guilford Press; 2020.
8. Kaye WH, Bulik CM, Thornton L, Barbarich N, Masters K. Comorbidity of anxiety disorders with anorexia and bulimia nervosa. Am J Psychiatry. 2004;161(12):2215–21. https://doi.org/10.1176/appi.ajp.161.12.2215.
9. Schaumberg K, Zerwas S, Goodman E, Yilmaz Z, Bulik CM, Micali N. Anxiety disorder symptoms at age 10 predict eating disorder symptoms and diagnoses in adolescence. J Child Psychol Psychiatry. 2018;60:686. https://doi.org/10.1111/jcpp.12984.
10. Godart NT, Flament MF, Lecrubier Y, Jeammet P. Anxiety disorders in anorexia nervosa and bulimia nervosa: co-morbidity and chronology of appearance. Eur Psychiatry. 2000;15(1):38–45. https://doi.org/10.1016/s0924-9338(00)00212-1.
11. Swinbourne JM, Touyz SW. The co-morbidity of eating disorders and anxiety disorders: a review. Eur Eat Disord Rev. 2007;15(4):253–74. https://doi.org/10.1002/erv.784.
12. American Psychiatric Association. Diagnostic and statistical manual of mental disorders, (DSM-5). Arlington: American Psychiatric Publishing; 2013.
13. Garner DM, Bemis KM. A cognitive-behavioral approach to anorexia nervosa. Cognit Ther Res. 1982;6(2):123–50. https://doi.org/10.1007/bf01183887.
14. Crisp A. Anorexia nervosa as flight from growth: assessment and treatment based on the model. In: Garner D, Garfinkel PE, editors. Handbook of treatment for eating disorders. New York: Guilford Press; 1997. p. 248–77.
15. Craske MG, Treanor M, Conway CC, Zbozinek T, Vervliet B. Maximizing exposure therapy: an inhibitory learning approach. Behav Res Ther. 2014;58:10–23. https://doi.org/10.1016/j.brat.2014.04.006.
16. Reilly EE, Anderson LM, Gorrell S, Schaumberg K, Anderson DA. Expanding exposure-based interventions for eating disorders. Int J Eat Disord. 2017;50(10):1137–41. https://doi.org/10.1002/eat.22761.
17. Bemis KM. A comparison of functional elationships in anorexia nervosa and phobia. In: Darby PL, Garfinkel PE, Garner DM, Coscina DV, editors. Anorexia nervosa: recent developments in research. New York: Allan R. Liss; 1983. p. 403–15.
18. Garner DM, Dalle Grave R. Terapia cognitivo comportamentale dei disturbi dell'alimentazione. Verona: Positive Press; 1999.
19. Dalle Grave R, Sartirana M, Calugi S. Weight phobia or overvaluation of shape and weight? A cognitive analysis of the core psychopathology of anorexia nervosa. IJEDO. 2019; https://doi.org/10.32044/ijedo.2019.08.

20. Fairburn CG, Cooper Z, Shafran R. Cognitive behaviour therapy for eating disorders: a "transdiagnostic" theory and treatment. Behav Res Ther. 2003;41(5):509–28. https://doi.org/10.1016/s0005-7967(02)00088-8.
21. Fairburn CG. Cognitive behavior therapy and eating disorders. New York: Guilford Press; 2008.
22. Godart NT, Flament MF, Perdereau F, Jeammet P. Comorbidity between eating disorders and anxiety disorders: a review. Int J Eat Disord. 2002;32(3):253–70. https://doi.org/10.1002/eat.10096.
23. Halmi KA, Tozzi F, Thornton LM, Crow S, Fichter MM, Kaplan AS, et al. The relation among perfectionism, obsessive-compulsive personality disorder and obsessive-compulsive disorder in individuals with eating disorders. Int J Eat Disord. 2005;38(4):371–4. https://doi.org/10.1002/eat.20190.
24. Sallet PC, de Alvarenga PG, Ferrao Y, de Mathis MA, Torres AR, Marques A, et al. Eating disorders in patients with obsessive-compulsive disorder: prevalence and clinical correlates. Int J Eat Disord. 2010;43(4):315–25. https://doi.org/10.1002/eat.20697.
25. Dalle Grave R, Calugi S, Marchesini G. Compulsive exercise to control shape or weight in eating disorders: prevalence, associated features, and treatment outcome. Compr Psychiatry. 2008;49(4):346–52. https://doi.org/10.1016/j.comppsych.2007.12.007.
26. Dalle Grave R. Features and management of compulsive exercising in eating disorders. Phys Sportsmed. 2009;37(3):20–8. https://doi.org/10.3810/psm.2009.10.1725.
27. Jacobi C, Hayward C, de Zwaan M, Kraemer HC, Agras WS. Coming to terms with risk factors for eating disorders: application of risk terminology and suggestions for a general taxonomy. Psychol Bull. 2004;130(1):19–65. https://doi.org/10.1037/0033-2909.130.1.19.
28. Brewerton TD. Eating disorders, trauma, and comorbidity: focus on PTSD. Eat Disord. 2007;15(4):285–304. https://doi.org/10.1080/10640260701454311.
29. Dansky BS, Brewerton TD, Kilpatrick DG, O'Neil PM. The National Women's study: relationship of victimization and posttraumatic stress disorder to bulimia nervosa. Int J Eat Disord. 1997;21(3):213–28. https://doi.org/10.1002/(sici)1098-108x(199704)21:3<213::aid-eat2>3.0.co;2-n.
30. Mitchell KS, Mazzeo SE, Schlesinger MR, Brewerton TD, Smith BN. Comorbidity of partial and subthreshold ptsd among men and women with eating disorders in the national comorbidity survey-replication study. Int J Eat Disord. 2012;45(3):307–15. https://doi.org/10.1002/eat.20965.
31. Calugi S, Franchini C, Pivari S, Conti M, El Ghoch M, Dalle Grave R. Anorexia nervosa and childhood sexual abuse: treatment outcomes of intensive enhanced cognitive behavioural therapy. Psychiatry Res. 2018;262(262):477–81. https://doi.org/10.1016/j.psychres.2017.09.027.
32. Bulik CM, Klump KL, Thornton L, Kaplan AS, Devlin B, Fichter MM, et al. Alcohol use disorder comorbidity in eating disorders: a multicenter study. J Clin Psychiatry. 2004;65(7):1000–6. https://doi.org/10.4088/jcp.v65n0718.
33. Root TL, Pisetsky EM, Thornton L, Lichtenstein P, Pedersen NL, Bulik CM. Patterns of co-morbidity of eating disorders and substance use in Swedish females. Psychol Med. 2010;40(1):105–15. https://doi.org/10.1017/s0033291709005662.

Chapter 7
Physical Complications

No physical examination or laboratory tests are required to make a diagnosis of eating disorders. Indeed, such a diagnosis is based solely on specific behavioural and attitudinal features, which must be detected by analysing the patients' history and examining their mental state [1]. However, patients with eating disorders, in particular those with anorexia nervosa or severe forms of bulimia nervosa, often present several, and in some cases severe, physical ailments that require accurate medical assessment and targeted management.

The physical anomalies observed in patients with eating disorders are in most cases secondary to a low-calorie diet, weight loss, purging behaviours (i.e. self-induced vomiting, misuse of laxatives and diuretics), and/or excessive exercising (see Chap. 2, Table 2.2) [2]. Most of these issues are fully resolved by restoration of adequate nutrition and a healthy weight. This indicates that, in general, but with a few exceptions, managing a patient's physical health should be focused on treating the eating disorder [1]. However, some clinical issues deserve particular mention, and may require additional, specific treatments. This chapter describes the management of the most common physical ailments encountered in eating disorders, and one clinical case with severe medical complications that was treated successfully in a specialist eating disorder unit.

7.1 Osteopenia and Osteoporosis

The onset of anorexia nervosa often coincides with the period of bone development, when people have not yet reached peak bone mass (which usually occurs between 17 and 22 years), and it is generally associated with amenorrhoea [3]. If adolescents with anorexia nervosa do not restore their body weight rapidly, the deposition of bone is compromised, leading to the development of permanent osteoporosis, which will increase the risk of fractures later in life [4]. Significant loss of bone mass,

R. Dalle Grave et al., *Complex Cases and Comorbidity in Eating Disorders*, https://doi.org/10.1007/978-3-030-69341-1_7

which can also continue or occur in adulthood, can be detected after just 6 months of weight loss, and is almost always present if the BMI is lower than 15.0.

The cause of bone loss in anorexia nervosa, as opposed to that which occurs in post-menopausal women, is multifactorial, and includes not only low oestrogen but also hypercortisolaemia, and reduced levels of androgens, leptin and insulin-like growth factor 1 (IGF-1). One of our studies found that in women with anorexia nervosa and amenorrhoea, bone resorption is elevated while bone formation is relatively depressed [5]. The consequence of this dynamic is that bone loss in anorexia nervosa is more severe than that occurring after menopause, where only bone resorption rate is raised.

The increase in bone resorption might provide a rationale for the use of antiresorptive drugs in patients with anorexia nervosa. However, the efficacy of oestrogen therapy is known to be poor, despite a slight increase in bone mineral density (BMD) having been reported after administration of physiological transdermal oestrogen replacement associated with weight regain in not severely underweight adolescents with anorexia nervosa [6]. Although evidence supporting its efficacy is weak, oestrogen therapy is commonly and ineffectively prescribed in patients with anorexia nervosa, with the risk of giving a false sense of normalcy [7].

Increases in spine BMD have been reported with bisphosphonate therapy [8]. However, bisphosphonates are not indicated for use in women of childbearing age, as it remains in the body for many years after discontinuation, and could have adverse effects on foetal development during pregnancy [7].

Other drugs tested for their potential effect of stimulating bone formation and mineralization, such as calcitonin, raloxifene and testosterone, have shown no positive effects in female patients with anorexia nervosa [7]. A study found that teriparatide does increase bone formation and BMD in women with anorexia nervosa [9], but its use is unrealistic due to its high cost, the label limitation regarding age, and that should be administered for no more than 24 months.

In the absence of drugs able to selectively suppress bone resorption without affecting bone formation, body weight restoration remains the cornerstone for treatment of bone disease in anorexia nervosa. Indeed, after weight gain an increase in body mass density does seem to occur in adult, as well as adolescent, women with anorexia nervosa. In fact, in one study we found that after 3 months of inpatient CBT-E and an increase in mean body weight from 37.8 to 51.5 kg, 55 consecutive women with anorexia had a significant mean increase in BMD, with percentage increases two- to threefold larger at the hip (2.6%) than at the spine (1.1%) [10].

We have also found that vitamin D status plays an important role and has implications for bone health in patients with anorexia nervosa. In the first of our studies, we discovered that vitamin D deficiency was widespread in a large cohort ($n = 89$) of untreated patients with anorexia nervosa and amenorrhoea: 16.9% had 25OH vitamin D levels below 12 ng/mL, 36% below 20 ng/mL, and 58.4% below 30 ng/mL (normal values $\geq$30 ng/mL) [11]. Moreover, we found a strong relationship between vitamin D status and hip BMD values, with additional benefits for those with 25OH vitamin D levels above 20 ng/mL [11]. In a second study, we evaluated BMD values in 91 consecutive female patients with anorexia nervosa treated via inpatient CBT-E for 20 weeks [12]. Although weight and BMI significantly increased in all patients during treatment, mean BMD increased only at the spine. The increase in spinal BMD was significantly higher only in those who had post-treatment 25OH vitamin D levels of above 30 ng/mL. In addition, we found a significant increase in parathormone (PTH), which was inversely correlated with decreased post-treatment 25OH vitamin D levels. This data led us to conclude that vitamin D deficiency may counteract the efficacy of refeeding through increased bone resorption mediated by secondary hyperparathyroidism, which strongly supports the use of vitamin D supplements for bone health in anorexia nervosa.

Finally, a systematic review by our team to assess the data on the association between weight gain/restoration and BMD in adolescents with anorexia nervosa concluded that weight gain is an effective strategy for promoting BMD increase in adolescents with anorexia nervosa. However, this process is slow, and improvements do not become detectable until approximately 16 months after weight restoration [13].

7.2 Amenorrhoea and Infertility

Primary or secondary amenorrhoea, although no longer considered a diagnostic criterion of anorexia nervosa [14], is a pathognomonic physical anomaly of this disorder. It is also called "functional hypothalamic amenorrhea"—a condition caused by stress, weight loss, and/or excessive exercising and characterized by cessation of the menstrual cycle due to dysfunction of the hypothalamic-pituitary-gonadal axis, abnormalities in gonadotropin pulsatility, and subsequent oestrogen deficiency [15]. Although secondary amenorrhoea may be the presenting manifestation of anorexia nervosa [16], it is strongly related to the loss of body weight [7].

Hence, weight restoration is the mainstay of treatment for secondary amenorrhea [7]. That being said, there is some disagreement about the degree of weight restoration needed for the resumption of normal periods, with some studies reporting the return of menstruation with the achievement of 90% of ideal body weight [17], and others with the body weight at which menstruation ceased [18].

The induction of menstruation with pharmacological intervention in underweight patients with anorexia nervosa is not indicated. Indeed, no clinical benefit has been found with the use of oestrogen replacement in these patients [19]. Moreover, as already stated in Sect. 7.1, the induction of withdrawal bleeding can give the patients a false sense of normality and, thereby, could reduce the motivation to change [7].

Since women with functional hypothalamic amenorrhea have low levels of leptin (a hormone secreted by fat cells correlated with the percentage of body fat and having a key role in regulating food intake and the hypothalamic–gonadal axis) [20], the administration of leptin to address the disrupted hypothalamic-gonadal axis has been researched. Two studies showed that recombinant leptin can restore the function of the hypothalamic-gonadal axis, leading to the resumption of menses [21, 22]. However, the participants in that study were normal weight, and leptin treatment has limited applicability in people with anorexia nervosa.

Provided that menstruation resumes, fertility is not compromised [23]. Nonetheless, despite a high prevalence of menstrual irregularities, women with anorexia nervosa have a higher risk of unplanned pregnancy than women without eating disorders [24]. Furthermore, although eating disorder psychopathology may remit during pregnancy, it often reappears after partum with rapid post-partum weight loss [24]. Finally, women with severe eating disorder symptoms prior to pregnancy more frequently have lower gestational weight, increased rate of caesarean partum, and babies with lower birthweight than women without anorexia nervosa [24].

7.3 Fluid and Electrolyte Abnormalities

The fluid and electrolyte abnormalities seen in patients with eating disorders are mainly the consequences of self-induced vomiting and/or misuse of laxatives and diuretics. These behaviours typically cause hypokalaemia and metabolic alkalosis, although in some cases a non-anion gap acidosis can be observed as a result of diarrhoea from laxative misuse [7].

The management of severe hypokalaemic metabolic alkalosis requires a medical intervention that is detailed and well described in previous publications [7, 25]. In most cases, hypokalaemia can be corrected orally but, when the serum level potassium falls below 2.5 mmol/L, it is preferable to administer potassium chloride intravenously [25]. Naturally, potassium supplementation should be associated with the suspension of purging behaviours and adequate hydration. Indeed, dehydration secondary to purging stimulates the secretion of aldosterone, which causes metabolic alkalosis and increases renal potassium excretion.

Other electrolyte disturbances that may require a correction are severe hyponatremia, which can also be the consequence of dehydration due to purging behaviours, excessive water intake and/or excessive exercising [26]. These behaviours may also cause hypochloraemia, hypophosphatemia, hypomagnesemia and/or decreased serum bicarbonate.

It is important to monitor and potentially treat patients who abruptly stop purging, as this can result in pseudo-Bartter's syndrome-induced oedema formation, and rapid weight gain due to the onset of oedema. Patients should be educated about this possibility and, in selected cases, treated with low-dose spironolactone for a couple of weeks [7]. In contrast, salt restriction is not indicated as it tends to increase aldosterone secretion and perpetuate oedema [7].

7.4   Cardiovascular Abnormalities

Eating disorders are associated with several cardiovascular complications, including haemodynamic issues, conduction disorders, and structural heart alterations. Although it is important to assess for and recognize these, in most cases they are completely reversible when weight is restored [7].

The most common hemodynamic alteration seen in eating disorders is hypotension (orthostatic or relative). Some authors recommend treatment with intravenous fluids if hypotension is symptomatic [7], but it generally requires no treatment as it completely resolves with a healthy diet and weight restoration.

The most common conduction system alteration of anorexia nervosa is bradycardia, but this too usually requires no pharmacological intervention. However, when patients present a persistent junctional rhythm (i.e. impulses coming from a tissue locus in the area of the atrioventricular node, the "junction" between the atria and ventricle), they should be monitored via telemetry [7], and potentially treadmill testing, to see if there is the conversion to sinus rhythm [27]. Another conduction alteration is QTc interval prolongation. This is usually associated with hypokalaemia secondary to purging behaviours. In these cases, patients should be monitored via electrocardiograms and telemetry, and treated with potassium and magnesium. It is also important to discontinue drugs that can prolong QTc intervals, such as neuroleptics and anti-emetics.

Reduction of left ventricular mass is the most common structural heart alteration in patients with anorexia nervosa [28], but this too is completely reversible through weight restoration [7]. Other alterations include pericardial effusion and mitral valve prolapse, which should be monitored but do not usually require any adjunctive treatment over nutritional rehabilitation and weight restoration. Finally, asymptomatic myocardial fibrosis has been found in 23% of patients with anorexia nervosa, leading to the speculation that this might be one of the reasons for the propensity of such individuals for sudden cardiac death [28].

7.5   Gastrointestinal Abnormalities

Delayed gastric emptying is common in underweight patients with eating disorder, and is associated with abdominal pain and bloating, especially after eating [29]. Such symptoms may create an obstacle to nutritional rehabilitation, and contribute to the maintenance of dietary restraint and restriction. Weight restoration usually improves gastric emptying [30], but low doses of metoclopramide can be prescribed to some patients who report extreme early satiation and feelings of fullness.

Constipation is the other gastrointestinal symptom frequently reported by patients with eating disorders. Indeed, constipation is often the result of reduced colonic motility secondary to dietary restriction and/or the misuse of laxatives. Constipation may also contribute to the maintenance of eating disorder psychopathology as some patients reduce their food intake as a means of alleviating it. Colonic motility improves with weight restoration and adequate fluid intake, but in some cases patients need to be encouraged to address constipation with osmotic laxatives, such as polyethene glycol powder and lactulose. Stimulant laxatives should not be used because they increase the risk of abdominal cramps and tend to damage colonic nerve cells in the long term [7].

Acid reflux is common in patients with self-induced vomiting, and should be treated with proton pump inhibitors. If patients are refractory to medical treatment or present dysphagia or a history of recurrent haematemesis, it is advisable to prescribe an upper endoscopy to exclude Barrett's oesophagus or oesophageal carcinoma (even though there is no data indicating that patients with eating disorders are at a higher risk of developing this type of cancer) [7].

Dental damage consequent to self-induced vomiting should be preventable with good dental hygiene to reduce the effect of stomach acid erosion of tooth enamel. Comprehensive dental procedures should not be undertaken until a significant reduction in self-induced vomiting has occurred [31]. Sialoadenosis, which in some cases may be the consequence of abrupt cessation of self-induced vomiting, can be managed with heat packs applied to the sides of the face and anti-inflammatory agents such as ibuprofen [7]. In rare refractory cases, pilocarpine may be tried before resorting to surgical treatment.

Other gastrointestinal abnormalities requiring medical treatment are haemorrhoids, and, more rarely, rectal prolapse—also a consequence of malnutrition and laxative misuse. Mesenteric artery syndrome is also a rare condition characterized by vomiting, abdominal pain, and further weight loss; it is due to compression of the third portion of the duodenum by the mesenteric plexus, caused by the loss of the adipose panicle. Some cases of acute gastric dilation, and more rarely stomach rupture, have been reported after binge-eating episodes. Violent self-induced vomiting may, albeit seldom, cause lacerations and bleeding to the wall of the oesophagus, and there is a remote risk of oesophageal rupture—a phenomenon which, like gastric rupture, is to be considered a medical emergency. We have also reported a solitary case of rectal ulcer syndrome in a patient with anorexia nervosa, which partially remitted after weight restoration [32].

Finally, an increase in liver enzymes may necessitate hospitalization but, in our clinical experience, these return rapidly to normal levels with refeeding, weight regain [33], and resting.

7.6   Clinical Issues Requiring Prompt Medical Intervention

A consensus document commissioned by the Italian Ministry of Health to indicate interventions for the intake, triage, assessment and treatment of patients with feeding and eating disorders has been developed by a group of Italian experts in the field [34]. The document outlines the main medical complications of eating disorders, and describes in detail the severity specifiers of such patients' physical state.

Table 7.1 Checklist of the main causes of clinical risk for patients with feeding and eating disorders who access emergency care [34, 35]

Significant clinical risk factors
• BMI <13 in adult patients (over 18 years of age) or <70% of the median paediatric BMI-for-age percentiles (in those under 18 years of age)
• Recent loss of more than 1 kg of body weight over a period of at least 2 consecutive weeks
• Recent history of poor or no nutrition for a period of at least 5 consecutive days.
• Fasting (refusal to intake food) or daily intake <500 kcal for a period of 2 days or more in a patient under the age of 18
• Habitual and recurrent self-induced vomiting or other purging behaviours (misuse of laxatives and/or diuretics)
• Heart rate <40 bpm
• Low systemic blood pressure values. Evidence of orthostatic hypotension (collapse of systolic blood pressure of 20 mmHg and/or of diastolic blood pressure of 10 mmHg within 3 min from the transition from supine to standing position). Presence of postural vertigo.
• Body temperature <35 °C
• Na <130 mmol/L or K <3.0 mmol/L
• Elevated transaminases
• Fasting blood glucose <3 mmol/L
• Increased urea or creatinine
• ECG anomalies, e.g. bradycardia; QTc >450 ms

Table 7.1 is derived from this consensus document [34], and from the recommendations of the MARSIPAN working group [35]; it takes into account the clinical risk elements of greatest importance, and may be used as a quick reference for emergency clinical assessment of patients with an eating disorder.

Vignette
The patient is a 28-year-old woman with anorexia nervosa. Her eating problem began at the age of 22 years, when she had a body weight of 48 kg (BMI 18.9), after she was left by her boyfriend and lost her job. She began to attend a gym daily, and the increased physical activity was associated with a non-intentional weight loss of about 2 kg in 1 month. This was accompanied by increased attention to the shape of her body, in particular her legs. Her preoccupation with her shape was associated with a further increase in the time spent in the gym, and the adoption of an extreme and rigid low-calorie diet. This produced a rapid weight loss, and the onset of secondary amenorrhea once her body weight fell to 44 kg. In 6 months she reached her lowest weight of 28 kg.

In the following 2 years, the patient was admitted four times to medical units to stabilize her medical conditions. She also received several specialist outpatient eating disorder treatments without obtaining a significant increase in body weight or improvement in eating disorder psychopathology. After 4 months of hospitalization in a specialist inpatient eating disorder unit, she normalized her body weight and maintained a BMI of about 19.0 for 3 consecutive years after discharge. However, she also maintained an extreme fear of weight gain, and, in the 6 months before consultation, after a slight increase in body weight, she adopted a strict and extreme low-calorie diet. This produced a weight loss of 12 kg, and she was referred us by her general practitioner.

After two assessment sessions, the patient agreed to be admitted to our inpatient CBT-E eating disorder unit, and at admission had a body weight of 39 kg (BMI 15.0). Dual-energy X-ray absorptiometry showed the presence of osteopenia (*t* score − 1.9) at the femur, while a blood test showed lows level of ferritin, haemoglobin and vitamin D.

One week after admission, the patient reported slight pain in the buttock, perineal and thigh regions, and an inability to climb the stairs. Pelvic X-ray showed an irregular, thin fissure at the level of the right ischiopubic ramus, indicating a non-displaced fracture (Fig. 7.1a). The consultant orthopaedic specialist recommended rest (lying down) to promote fracture healing. After this recommendation, the patient became even more uncooperative, refusing to lie down or eat the planned meals, using her inability to walk (as she had been able to do before the fracture) to justify her decision. This behaviour produced a weight loss of 1 kg in 1 week and was associated with deterioration in both her medical conditions and eating disorder psychopathology.

Thereafter, the main focus of the intervention was therefore on motivating the patient to take an active part in addressing her eating disorder psychopathology, and agreeing to rest, which would be vital to promote fracture healing. To achieve these goals, the team used specific CBT-E engagement strategies. The patient was helped to choose to accept rest and interrupt her excessive exercising, rather than imposing the decision on her. After two sessions, the patient reached the conclusion that the

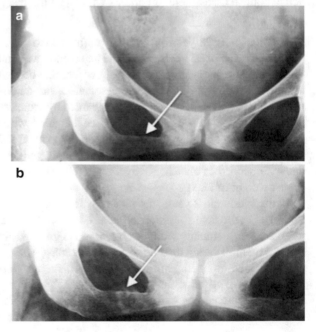

Fig. 7.1 Plain radiograph showing (**a**) non-displaced stress fracture with (**b**) callus formation at the inferior ischiopubic ramus in a 28-year-old woman with anorexia nervosa **From El Ghoch M, Bazzani P, Dalle Grave R. Management of ischiopubic stress fracture in patients with anorexia nervosa and excessive compulsive exercising. BMJ Case Rep. 2014;2014. doi:https://doi. org/10.1136/ bcr-2014-206393. Reprinted with the permission of BMJ Publishing Group Ltd**

positive aspects of excessive exercising are of brief duration and invariably associated with negative emotions (e.g. guilt if an exercise session is missed), and, in this case, with a high risk of poor recovery from the pelvic stress fracture. To address the patient's fear of uncontrolled weight gain (as a result of resting), the patient was informed that the adoption of healthy eating and exercising is the optimal strategy to maintain weight control in the long term. Moreover, changing her unhealthy exercising practice would be a positive opportunity for a new start, a life no longer conditioned by the need to exercise. Since the patient remained reluctant, we suggest to her that she "take the plunge" and make a fresh start on a trial basis. We also informed her that in the first few days her anxiety levels and concerns about shape and weight would be likely to increase, but that these would gradually fade away as the treatment progressed.

These procedures helped the patient to address her urge to exercise, and to follow the recommendation of the orthopaedic specialist. The patient gradually became actively engaged in the treatment, resting as recommended, and X-ray at 35 days (Fig. 7.1b) showed complete fracture healing. After a total of 20 weeks (13 inpatient and 7 day-hospital), the patient was discharged with a body weight of 47.5 kg (BMI 18.8). Following discharge, the patient completed a 6-month outpatient CBT-E programme, and at 12 months follow-up had a body weight of 51 kg (BMI 20.1), regular menses, complete remission of the eating disorder psychopathology, good social relationships, and a job as an au pair.

Two clinical considerations can be derived from this case report [36]. First is the need to pay special attention in patients with anorexia nervosa, even if they are not osteoporotic, to the possible development of pelvic fracture when they present other risk factors for stress fractures, such as excessive exercising, low serum levels of vitamin D, iron deficiency and amenorrhoea. Second, in these patients, specific CBT-E strategies and procedures used to treat the eating disorder psychopathology can be successfully adapted to encourage rest, without adopting coercive measures.

References

1. Fairburn CG, Harrison PJ. Eating disorders. Lancet. 2003;361(9355):407–16. https://doi.org/10.1016/s0140-6736(03)12378-1.
2. Dalle Grave R, Calugi S. Cognitive behavior therapy for adolescents with eating disorders. New York: Guilford Press; 2020.
3. Misra M, Klibanski A. Endocrine consequences of anorexia nervosa. Lancet Diabetes Endocrinol. 2014;2(7):581–92. https://doi.org/10.1016/s2213-8587(13)70180-3.
4. Lucas AR, Melton LJ 3rd, Crowson CS, O'Fallon WM. Long-term fracture risk among women with anorexia nervosa: a population-based cohort study. Mayo Clin Proc. 1999;74(10):972–7. https://doi.org/10.4065/74.10.972.
5. Idolazzi L, El Ghoch M, Dalle Grave R, Bazzani PV, Calugi S, Fassio S, et al. Bone metabolism in patients with anorexia nervosa and amenorrhoea. Eat Weight Disord. 2016; https://doi.org/10.1007/s40519-016-0337-x.

6. Misra M, Katzman D, Miller KK, Mendes N, Snelgrove D, Russell M, et al. Physiologic estrogen replacement increases bone density in adolescent girls with anorexia nervosa. J Bone Miner Res. 2011;26(10):2430–8. https://doi.org/10.1002/jbmr.447.

7. Mehler PS, Krantz MJ, Sachs KV. Treatments of medical complications of anorexia nervosa and bulimia nervosa. J Eat Disord. 2015;3:15. https://doi.org/10.1186/s40337-015-0041-7.

8. Miller KK, Meenaghan E, Lawson EA, Misra M, Gleysteen S, Schoenfeld D, et al. Effects of risedronate and low-dose transdermal testosterone on bone mineral density in women with anorexia nervosa: a randomized, placebo-controlled study. J Clin Endocrinol Metab. 2011;96(7):2081–8. https://doi.org/10.1210/jc.2011-0380.

9. Fazeli PK, Wang IS, Miller KK, Herzog DB, Misra M, Lee H, et al. Teriparatide increases bone formation and bone mineral density in adult women with anorexia nervosa. J Clin Endocrinol Metab. 2014;99(4):1322–9. https://doi.org/10.1210/jc.2013-4105.

10. Viapiana O, Gatti D, Dalle Grave R, Todesco T, Rossini M, Braga V, et al. Marked increases in bone mineral density and biochemical markers of bone turnover in patients with anorexia nervosa gaining weight. Bone. 2007;40(4):1073–7. https://doi.org/10.1016/j.bone.2006.11.015.

11. Gatti D, El Ghoch M, Viapiana O, Ruocco A, Chignola E, Rossini M, et al. Strong relationship between vitamin D status and bone mineral density in anorexia nervosa. Bone. 2015;78:212–5. https://doi.org/10.1016/j.bone.2015.05.014.

12. Giollo A, Idolazzi L, Caimmi C, Fassio A, Bertoldo F, Dalle Grave R, et al. Vitamin D levels strongly influence bone mineral density and bone turnover markers during weight gain in female patients with anorexia nervosa. Int J Eat Disord. 2017;50(9):1041–9. https://doi.org/10.1002/eat.22731.

13. El Ghoch M, Gatti D, Calugi S, Viapiana O, Bazzani PV, Dalle Grave R. The association between weight gain/restoration and bone mineral density in adolescents with anorexia nervosa: a systematic review. Nutrients. 2016;8(12). https://doi.org/10.3390/nu8120769.

14. American Psychiatric Association. Diagnostic and statistical manual of mental disorders, (DSM-5). Arlington: American Psychiatric Publishing; 2013.

15. Gordon CM, Ackerman KE, Berga SL, Kaplan JR, Mastorakos G, Misra M, et al. Functional hypothalamic amenorrhea: an Endocrine Society clinical practice guideline. J Clin Endocrinol Metab. 2017;102(5):1413–39. https://doi.org/10.1210/jc.2017-00131.

16. Dalle Grave R, Calugi S, Marchesini G. Is amenorrhea a clinically useful criterion for the diagnosis of anorexia nervosa? Behav Res Ther. 2008;46(12):1290–4. https://doi.org/10.1016/j.brat.2008.08.007.

17. Golden NH, Jacobson MS, Schebendach J, Solanto MV, Hertz SM, Shenker IR. Resumption of menses in anorexia nervosa. Arch Pediatr Adolesc Med. 1997;151(1):16–21. https://doi.org/10.1001/archpedi.1997.02170380020003.

18. Swenne I. Weight requirements for return of menstruations in teenage girls with eating disorders, weight loss and secondary amenorrhoea. Acta Paediatr. 2004;93(11):1449–55. https://doi.org/10.1080/08035250410033303.

19. Bergström I, Crisby M, Engström AM, Hölcke M, Fored M, Jakobsson Kruse P, et al. Women with anorexia nervosa should not be treated with estrogen or birth control pills in a bone-sparing effect. Acta Obstet Gynecol Scand. 2013;92(8):877–80. https://doi.org/10.1111/aogs.12178.

20. Warren MP, Voussoughian F, Geer EB, Hyle EP, Adberg CL, Ramos RH. Functional hypothalamic amenorrhea: Hypoleptinemia and disordered eating. J Clin Endocrinol Metab. 1999;84(3):873–7. https://doi.org/10.1210/jcem.84.3.5551.

21. Welt CK, Chan JL, Bullen J, Murphy R, Smith P, DePaoli AM, et al. Recombinant human leptin in women with hypothalamic amenorrhea. N Engl J Med. 2004;351(10):987–97. https://doi.org/10.1056/NEJMoa040388.

22. Sienkiewicz E, Magkos F, Aronis KN, Brinkoetter M, Chamberland JP, Chou S, et al. Long-term metreleptin treatment increases bone mineral density and content at the lumbar spine of lean hypoleptinemic women. Metabolism. 2011;60(9):1211–21. https://doi.org/10.1016/j.metabol.2011.05.016.

23. Bulik CM, Sullivan PF, Fear JL, Pickering A, Dawn A, McCullin M. Fertility and reproduction in women with anorexia nervosa: a controlled study. J Clin Psychiatry. 1999;60(2):130–5; quiz 5–7. https://doi.org/10.4088/jcp.v60n0212.
24. Hoffman ER, Zerwas SC, Bulik CM. Reproductive issues in anorexia nervosa. Expert Rev Obstet Gynecol. 2011;6(4):403–14. https://doi.org/10.1586/eog.11.31.
25. Mehler PS, Andersen AE. Eating disorders: a guide to medical care and complications. 3nd ed. Baltimore: Johns Hopkins University Press; 2017.
26. El Ghoch M, Calugi S, Dalle Grave R. Management of severe rhabdomyolysis and exercise-associated hyponatremia in a female with anorexia nervosa and excessive compulsive exercising. Case Rep Med. 2016;2016:8194160. https://doi.org/10.1155/2016/8194160.
27. Krantz MJ, Gaudiani JL, Johnson VW, Mehler PS. Exercise electrocardiography extinguishes persistent junctional rhythm in a patient with severe anorexia nervosa. Cardiology. 2011;120(4):217–20. https://doi.org/10.1159/000335481.
28. Oflaz S, Yucel B, Oz F, Sahin D, Ozturk N, Yaci O, et al. Assessment of myocardial damage by cardiac MRI in patients with anorexia nervosa. Int J Eat Disord. 2013;46(8):862–6. https://doi.org/10.1002/eat.22170.
29. Kamal N, Chami T, Andersen A, Rosell FA, Schuster MM, Whitehead WE. Delayed gastrointestinal transit times in anorexia nervosa and bulimia nervosa. Gastroenterology. 1991;101(5):1320–4. https://doi.org/10.1016/0016-5085(91)90083-w.
30. Benini L, Todesco T, Dalle Grave R, Deiorio F, Salandini L, Vantini I. Gastric emptying in patients with restricting and binge/purging subtypes of anorexia nervosa. Am J Gastroenterol. 2004;99(8):1448–54. https://doi.org/10.1111/j.1572-0241.2004.30246.x.
31. Faine MP. Recognition and management of eating disorders in the dental office. Dent Clin N Am. 2003;47(2):395–410. https://doi.org/10.1016/s0011-8532(02)00108-8.
32. El Ghoch M, Benini L, Sgarbi D, Dalle Grave R. Solitary rectal ulcer syndrome in a patient with anorexia nervosa: a case report. Int J Eat Disord. 2016;49(7):731–5. https://doi.org/10.1002/eat.22548.
33. Rosen E, Bakshi N, Watters A, Rosen HR, Mehler PS. Hepatic complications of anorexia nervosa. Dig Dis Sci. 2017;62(11):2977–81. https://doi.org/10.1007/s10620-017-4766-9.
34. Ministero della Salute: Interventi per l'accoglienza, il triage, la valutazione ed il trattamento del paziente con disturbi della nutrizione e dell'alimentazione. Percorso lilla in pronto soccorso (Revisione 2020); 2020. http://www.salute.gov.it/portale/documentazione/p6_2_2_1.jsp?lingua=italiano&id=2961
35. Robinson P, Rhys JW. MARSIPAN: management of really sick patients with anorexia nervosa. BJPsych Adv. 2018;24(1):20–32. https://doi.org/10.1192/bja.2017.2.
36. El Ghoch M, Bazzani P, Dalle Grave R. Management of ischiopubic stress fracture in patients with anorexia nervosa and excessive compulsive exercising. BMJ Case Rep. 2014;2014. https://doi.org/10.1136/bcr-2014-206393.

Chapter 8
Coexisting General Medical Diseases

Eating disorders may coexist with a variety of general medical diseases. The most common medical comorbidity is obesity, although this is largely exclusively confined to patients with binge-eating disorder. The other most common general medical conditions that clinicians may observe in some patients with eating disorders are as follows: type 1 diabetes, coeliac disease, inflammatory bowel disease and irritable bowel syndrome. Some patients also report food allergies, which are, however, often ruled out by accurate diagnostic testing.

Therapists assessing a patient with an eating disorder coexisting with a general medical disease should keep the following questions in mind [1]:

- *Am I sufficiently expert in the general medical disease to appropriately assess and treat it?* The treatment of general medical disease must be conducted by medical doctors. However, we recommend that non-medical therapists educate themselves (e.g. consulting reliable websites) and ask medical colleagues for information about the general medical disease. It is also important that clinicians read the literature describing the coexistence of the two disorders.
- *Are the eating disorders and the general medical disease interacting, and, if so, in what way?* The therapist should assess whether there is an interaction between the two disorders and whether their coexistence is harmful.
- *Are the medical doctors who are treating the general medical disease aware of the eating disorder, and how it may impact the patient's health?* Patients should be always encouraged to inform their attending physician that they are in treatment for an eating disorder.
- *Are the features of the general medical disease or its treatment likely to complicate the treatment of the eating disorder, and* vice versa? If this seems to be the case, with the patient's consent it is advisable to discuss the nature of this interaction and the strategies adopted to manage the two disorders with their physician, and to address any potential obstacles that may arise.

R. Dalle Grave et al., *Complex Cases and Comorbidity in Eating Disorders*, https://doi.org/10.1007/978-3-030-69341-1_8

- *Does CBT-E need to be adapted to accommodate the general medical disorder?* In some cases, certain procedures (e.g. what to include in the self-monitoring records, and the dietary rules to address) may need to be adapted due to the coexistence of the general medical disease. It may also be necessary to adjust the duration of the standard treatment for eating disorder.

In this chapter, we describe the strategies for assessing and treating the main general medical diseases that coexist with eating disorder psychopathology.

8.1 Obesity

Obesity is the medical condition most frequently observed in people with eating disorders. It frequently coexists with binge-eating disorder, and with some cases of bulimia nervosa. Obesity can precede the onset of the eating disorder, sometimes representing a risk factor for its onset, or may be the consequence of recurrent episodes of binge-eating. Eating disorders and obesity, when they coexist, tend to interact negatively with each other and make treatment more problematic. Table 8.1 describes some general information about obesity for non-medical therapists.

Table 8.1 General information on obesity

Obesity is a chronic relapsing disease process [2] characterized by abnormal or excessive fat accumulation that may impair health [3].
BMI is used to classify overweight and obesity in adults, and is calculated as a person's weight in kilograms divided by the square of their height in metres (kg/m^2). Adults are defined as overweight when their BMI is between 25 and 29.9, while a BMI of 30 or more denotes obesity [3]. For children aged between 5 and 19 years, overweight and obesity are defined when their BMI-for-age percentile is greater than 1 and 2 standard deviations above the World Health Organization (WHO) growth reference median, respectively [3]. It should be noted, however, that although BMI is a useful population-level measure of overweight and obesity, it may not correspond to the same degree of "fatness" in different individuals.
Obesity is a complex disease caused by the interaction of genetic and environmental factors. Genetic factors seem to account for 40–70% of the cause [4], exacerbated by an obesogenic environment encouraging an increased intake of energy-dense foods that are high in fat and sugars, and an increase in sedentary behaviour [3]. Obesity can also stem from eating disorders, mainly binge-eating disorder [5], and some drugs that induce weight gain (e.g. antipsychotics, antidepressants, antiepileptics, insulin and insulin secretagogues, glucocorticoids, oral contraceptives, beta-blockers, and others) [6].
Obesity is associated with a higher risk of developing non-communicable diseases such as cardiovascular diseases (mainly heart disease and stroke), diabetes, musculoskeletal disorders (especially osteoarthritis—a highly disabling degenerative disease of the joints), and some cancers (including endometrial, breast, ovarian, prostate, liver, gallbladder, kidney, and colon) [3]. Obesity also impairs quality of life [7], is a significant risk factor for disability [8] and is associated with higher all-cause mortality [9]. Finally, there is strong negative association with weight bias internalization, which occurs when individuals apply negative societal weight-related stereotypes to themselves, and self-derogate because of their body weight. This may have a considerable impact on mental health [10].

8.1.1 Prevalence

Among seeking-treatment patients for obesity, 1.4–9% meet the DSM-5 diagnostic criteria for binge-eating disorder [11–13], although in the same population the presence of binge-eating episodes has been reported with a range of between 9 and 29% [11–13]. Patients with obesity and binge-eating disorder have a higher BMI than patients with obesity but not the disorder [11]. There is no reliable data on the prevalence of bulimia nervosa in obesity, but the coexistence of the two conditions does not seem to be very frequent.

8.1.2 Risk Factors

Case-controlled and cohort studies have revealed that pre-morbid and family obesity is a risk factor for both bulimia nervosa [14] and binge-eating disorder [15, 16]. It has been hypothesized that, in Western countries, obesity increases the risk of receiving critical comments about shape and weight from others, developing body dissatisfaction, and the adoption strict dieting, potentially increasing the risk of the eating disorder onset [17]. In particular, body-image risk factors may increase the probability of internalizing the "thin ideal",[1] accompanied by the development of overvaluation of shape and weight; the adoption of rigid and extreme dietary rules may be implicated in the onset of binge-eating episodes.

8.1.3 Interactions between Eating Disorders and Obesity

When they coexist, eating disorders and obesity interact negatively with each other through three main mechanisms [18]: (i) binge-eating episodes promote weight gain; (ii) excess weight increases concerns about body shape and weight and encourages the adoption of a strict diet and other extreme weight control behaviours which, in turn, increase the risk of binge-eating episodes; and (iii) excess weight is often associated with reduced physical activity levels and consequently an increased risk of having negative emotional states that can trigger binge-eating episodes.

8.1.4 Clinical Consequences

When obesity coexists with binge-eating disorder, it is characterized by a worsening of medical comorbidities and physical disability. A study based on self-reported data found that, after adjusting the data for age, sex, BMI and BMI interval change,

---

[1] The concept of the ideally slim (female) body.

individuals with binge-eating disorder have a greater frequency of new diagnoses of metabolic syndrome components (i.e. dyslipidaemia, hypertension, and type 2 diabetes) than those with no history of eating disorder [19].

The association between binge-eating disorder and a higher frequency of obesity-related medical comorbidities has been confirmed by studies that used a semi-structured interview and checked for potential confounders. For example, after adjusting the data for age, sex, education, BMI, and psychiatric/emotional health, binge-eating disorder was found to be linked to altered blood sugar levels, cardiovascular diseases and severe walking limitations [20]. These findings indicate that binge-eating disorder appears to confer an additional cardiometabolic risk, greater than that attributable to obesity alone.

It has been hypothesized that in people with binge-eating disorder, increased weight-independent medical comorbidities are likely to be the result of their unhealthy lifestyle, characterized by smoking, low levels of exercise, alcohol abuse and poor eating, with recurring binge-eating episodes involving eating foods high in fat, sugar and/or salt, but low in vitamins and minerals. This may explain why people with binge-eating disorder and obesity often suffer from both the typical complications associated with obesity (e.g. metabolic syndrome and type 2 diabetes) and other weight-independent medical problems such as irritable bowel syndrome, as well as complications related to alcohol abuse and smoking; neck, shoulder and lower back pain; and chronic muscle pain [21].

8.1.5   Is Weight Loss Indicated?

Weight loss is always contraindicated when obesity coexists with bulimia nervosa. Indeed, according to transdiagnostic cognitive behaviour theory [22], binge-eating episodes are largely maintained (as described in Chap. 3 Sect. 3.2) by the attempt to adhere to extreme and rigid eating rules and/or severe dietary restriction (i.e. undereating in physiological terms) (Fig. 6.1). People with bulimia nervosa tend to react in a negative and extreme, often dichotomous, way to the almost inevitable breaking of the dietary rules adopted for the purposes of losing weight. Even a small transgression tends to be interpreted as evidence of a lack of self-control, and results in temporary abandonment of the effort to restrict the diet, resulting in a binge-eating episode. This, in turn, maintains the overvaluation of shape and weight by intensifying concerns about being unable to control shape, weight and eating, and encourages further dietary restriction, thus increasing the risk of further binge-eating episodes. With this in mind, weight loss should only be considered in patients with obesity and bulimia nervosa after a prolonged period of remission from the eating disorder (at least 1 year) (Fig. 8.1).

When obesity coexists with binge-eating disorder, there is not an absolute contraindication to weight loss [23]. However, while the available treatments (e.g. CBT for eating disorders, interpersonal psychotherapy [IPT], CBT-based guided self-help, and pharmacological agents) are effective in reducing the frequency of

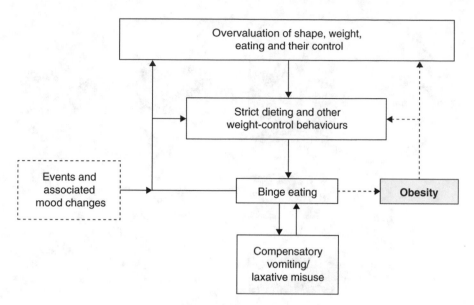

Fig. 8.1 Formulation of a patient with bulimia nervosa and coexisting obesity

binge-eating episodes, their impact on long-term weight loss in patients with episodes of binge-eating is poor [24, 25]. Furthermore, research has found that sequential treatment (behavioural weight loss followed by CBT for eating disorders) is not superior to CBT for eating disorders alone [26]. Other approaches have combined CBT for eating disorders with weight-loss drugs [27], dietetic interventions [28] or a physical activity programme [29], but yielded no clear results demonstrating their greater efficacy with respect to CBT alone. The presence of binge-eating disorder also seems to predict less weight loss and weight regain in patients with binge-eating disorder and obesity treated via bariatric surgery, especially in the subgroup of patients who have recurrent episodes of loss of control over eating, even though these are often characterized by the repeated intake of small amounts of food due to the anatomical limitations introduced by the intervention [30].

Recently we have proposed an innovative integrated treatment that addresses the two goals of cessation of binge-eating episodes and weight loss [18]. The treatment, described in detail in a previous publication [18] and currently under investigation, is based on a theoretical model of the factors that maintain both binge-eating episodes and the associated obesity/overweight (Fig. 8.2). Using this model, treatment can be personalized to address the key maintenance processes acting in the patient, thereby making it suitable for a variety of different clinical presentations of binge-eating disorder. The new integrated treatment is modular, and incorporates elements from CBT-E for eating disorders that have been shown to be effective in reducing binge eating [31], and CBT for obesity, a programme which produces a loss of 6.8% of initial body weight, with 71% of patients achieving a weight loss of ≥5%, as well as significant improvements in eating disorder psychopathology [32, 33]. In short,

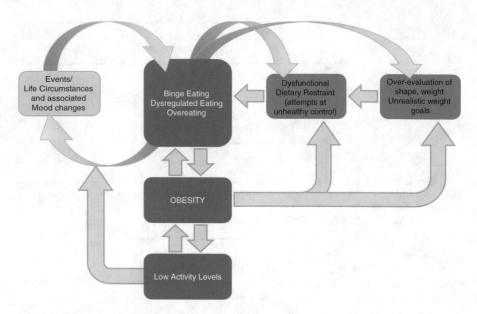

Fig. 8.2 Key maintenance processes of binge-eating disorder with coexisting obesity/overweight From Cooper, Z., Calugi, S., & Dalle Grave, R. (2019). Controlling binge eating and weight: A treatment for binge eating disorder worth researching? Eating and Weight Disorders. doi:https://doi.org/10.1007/s40519-019-00734-4. Reprinted with the permission of Springer Nature

patients are first helped to reduce binge-eating episodes via the CBT-E regular eating procedure (i.e. self-monitoring in real-time, eating three planned meals and two snacks and not eating between). Once this goal has been achieved, the treatment integrates the other CBT-E strategies and procedures to address the eating disorder psychopathology with a moderate and "flexible" low-calorie diet, associated with the adoption of an active lifestyle [23]. Indeed, the most recent research has confirmed that dietary restraint (i.e. the cognitive state involved in trying to adhere to dietary rules) is not a unitary concept [34], and that flexible, as opposed to rigid, dietary restraint is not inconsistent with controlling binge eating. In fact, such a flexible approach to eating is associated with both the remission of binge eating and better weight loss [35].

Vignette

The patient, a single 30-year-old woman with a BMI of 34.0, reported progressive weight gain from the age of 22, which could be linked to the onset of recurrent binge-eating episodes not followed by the adoption of compensatory behaviours. The binge-eating episodes had begun after the breakup of a relationship that had lasted for 4 years. The course of the eating disorder was characterized by the alternation of prolonged periods in which binge-eating episodes had a daily frequency and were associated with marked weight gain, and periods of strict dieting that resulted in a rapid weight loss, followed by a prolonged period of recurrent binge-eating episodes.

In the 3 months preceding consultation, the patient reported the presence of recurrent binge-eating episodes (five times a week on average), not followed by compensatory behaviours, in association with events and associated mood changes. The binge-eating episodes had the following features: eating much more rapidly than normal; eating until feeling uncomfortably full; and eating large amounts of food when not feeling physically hungry. Between binge-eating episodes, the patient reported dysregulated eating characterized by the absence of formal meals (she skipped breakfast and often also lunch) and the frequent intake of snacks and other high-calorie foods (biscuits, sweets, crisps, ice creams, etc.). After each binge-eating episode, the patient felt disgusted with herself, but although very dissatisfied with her body, did not seem to overvalue shape, weight and their control.

The therapist first educated the patient about the main processes maintaining binge-eating disorder and obesity, and how they interact with each other by drawing a personalized formulation similar to that illustrated in Fig. 8.2. The first 3 weeks of outpatient treatment were dedicated to implementing self-monitoring in real-time, weekly collaborative weighing, and reducing the frequency of binge-eating episodes via the regular eating procedure (see Chap. 3, Table 3.1). During this time the patient experienced only one binge-eating episode, which occurred in the last week and was triggered by an argument with her mother. Otherwise, she proved herself capable of eating three meals plus two snacks a day, without eating between them.

After reviewing with the therapist the previous failure of her weight loss attempts, which were characterized by the adoption of extreme and rigid dietary rules, the patient agreed to the therapist's proposal that she can follow a moderate but flexible dietary restriction regime (about 500 kcal less than she was consuming daily), associated with a progressive increase in the number of daily steps she was taking. At the same time, her treatment addressed residual binge-eating episodes with the strategies and procedures in the CBT-E Events, Moods and Eating module (see Chap. 3, Table 3.1).

After 6 months, the patient had achieved a 7% weight loss and complete remission of her binge-eating episodes. Although her weight loss was lower than she had expected at the beginning of the treatment, the patient was very satisfied with the results achieved and agreed to start the strategies and procedures for maintaining her body weight [23]. After 1 year of maintenance, her weight remained stable and the binge-eating disorder was in remission.

8.2 Type 1 Diabetes

The prevalence, clinical characteristics and medical consequences of eating disorders in people with type 1 diabetes have received increasing attention since reports of this dangerous combination were first published in the 1980s [36]. Although the specificity of this association was initially unclear, systematic research over the past two decades has shown that eating disorders are more common in people with type 1 diabetes than in the general population [37]. Current evidence indicates that the

Table 8.2 General information on type 1 diabetes

Type 1 diabetes is a chronic disease in which the beta cells of the pancreas produce very little or no insulin [40] due to autoimmune disease [41]. Insulin is a hormone needed to allow sugar (glucose) to enter cells and produce energy. Without treatment, insulin deficit results in high blood sugar levels and specific symptoms that typically develop over a short period of time, such as excess excretion of urine (polyuria), thirst (polydipsia), constant hunger, weight loss, vision changes and fatigue [41].

Type 1 diabetes may occur at any age, but its onset is typically between the ages of 4 and 6, or between 10 and 14. The cause of type 1 diabetes is unknown, although it seems to derive from a combination of genetic and environment factors, such as viral infection [42].

The diagnosis of diabetes is made by testing the level of sugar or glycated haemoglobin (HbA1C) in the blood, and type 1 diabetes can be distinguished from type 2 by testing for the presence of specific autoantibodies [43].

Treatment with insulin, given by injection under skin or via an insulin pump, is required to survive [42]. A healthy diet and exercise may improve the outcome of insulin treatment and help prevent complications [44].

Typical rapid onset complications include diabetic ketoacidosis, also known as diabetic coma—a life-threatening medical condition caused by the body's need to break down fats for energy instead of using sugars [41]. Long-term complications include cardiovascular disease, diabetic neuropathy and diabetic retinopathy [41]. Excessive doses of insulin can cause severe hypoglycaemia.

coexistence of eating disorder with type 1 diabetes is associated with poor glycaemic control, and a consequently higher risk of medical complications [38], while the presence of type 1 diabetes may contribute to the maintenance of the eating disorder psychopathology [39]. Table 8.2 provides some general information on type 1 diabetes for non-medical therapists.

8.2.1   Diagnostic Issues

Diagnosis of eating disorder in people with type 1 diabetes is difficult because patients tend to hide and deny the adoption of problematic eating behaviours [38]. In addition, the self-reported questionnaires used for the assessment of the psychopathology and prevalence of eating disorders are only partially appropriate for individuals with type 1 diabetes for two main reasons: (i) they do not identify certain eating disorder behaviours adopted by individuals with type 1 diabetes, such as the reduction or omission of insulin; and (ii) they tend to overestimate the prevalence of eating disorders because some behaviours considered disturbed (e.g. food concern, limiting the intake of certain food groups, and eating when not hungry) are an integral part of diabetes care.

In some studies, the 16-item Diabetes Eating Problem Survey-Revised (DEPS-R) tool [45] has been used to screen for the presence of "disordered eating", but not eating disorders. Indeed, although it measures eating behaviours and abnormal behaviours specific to individuals with type 1 diabetes (e.g. skipping next insulin dose after overeating, avoiding the measurement of blood sugar when thinking it is

Table 8.3 Warning signs that may point to the presence of an eating disorder in a patient with type 1 diabetes

- Unexplained increases in glycated haemoglobin (HbA1c)
- Repeated episodes of diabetic ketoacidosis due to insulin omission
- Extreme concerns about shape and weight
- Morbid fear of gaining weight
- Unexplained weight loss
- Low weight
- Avoiding measuring body weight or frequent weight checking
- Feeling fat
- Frequent and abnormal body checking
- Adoption of extreme and rigid dietary rules
- Recurrent binge-eating episodes
- Recurrent self-induced vomiting episodes
- Misuse of laxatives and/or diuretics
- Excessive exercising
- Secondary amenorrhea

beyond the appropriate range, trying to keep blood glucose high to lose weight, trying to eat to the point of expelling ketones in the urine), it does not include specific questions for assessing the core eating disorder psychopathology (i.e. the overvaluation of shape, weight, eating and their control).

Table 8.3 shows the main warning signs that may suggest that there is an eating disorder in a person with type 1 diabetes.

8.2.2   Prevalence

Prevalence rates for eating disorders in people with type 1 diabetes vary depending on the different diagnostic categories of eating disorders and the populations studied.

- *Anorexia nervosa, bulimia nervosa and eating disorders not otherwise specified* (global prevalence). A meta-analysis of six studies in adolescents found a higher prevalence rate of eating disorders in individuals with type 1 diabetes than in those without type 1 diabetes (7.0% vs. 2.8%, respectively) [37].
- *Anorexia nervosa.* A meta-analysis of controlled studies using the DSM-III or IV diagnostic criteria found no significant differences in the prevalence of anorexia nervosa in people with type 1 diabetes as compared to controls [46].

- *Bulimia nervosa.* The same meta-analysis found a higher prevalence of bulimia nervosa in women with type 1 diabetes than in controls [46]. To define the coexistence of these two conditions, some authors used the term "diabulimia" [47].
- *Disordered eating.* As evaluated by the DEPS-R [45], this category describes individuals who report disordered eating behaviours, but not necessarily an eating disorder of clinical severity. A meta-analysis of five studies found a higher prevalence of disordered eating in adolescents with type 1 diabetes than in controls (39.3% vs. 32.5%, respectively) [37]. The prevalence of disordered eating increased significantly with weight and age [48], from 7.2% in the underweight group to 32.7% in the group with obesity, and from 8.1% in the youngest age group (11–13 years) to 38.1% in the older age group (17–19 years). A recent study of 163 Italian adolescents (11–20 years of age) with type 1 diabetes found an incidence of disordered eating of 27% in boys and 42% in girls [49]. Participants with disordered eating had a clinical profile characterized by being overweight, devoting little time to physical activity, low socioeconomic status, poor metabolic control and a tendency to skip insulin injections.
- *Restriction or omission of insulin.* This is more frequent in females, and increases with age, affecting up to 40% of young adults with type 1 diabetes [38]. In some patients, the restriction or omission of insulin is used after objective binge-eating episodes, while in others it even occurs after normal meals—a condition that might be defined as "purging disorder" by the DSM-5 [50].

8.2.3   Risk Factors

Why there is an increased prevalence of eating disorders and disordered eating in individuals with type 1 diabetes is not known, although it appears to stem from a complex combination of genetic and environmental factors. The genetic link between eating disorders and diabetes is in part supported by the latest genome-wide association study that identified eight significant genome-wide loci for anorexia nervosa and significant genetic correlations with psychiatric disorders, physical activity, metabolic (including glycaemic), lipid, and anthropometric traits, independent of the effects of common variants associated with BMI [51]. Type 1 diabetes is also associated with some common eating disorder risk factors. For example, people with diabetes have twice the risk of clinical depression than those without [52], while girls with type 1 diabetes often have a higher BMI than their peers without diabetes [53].

The psychology literature has proposed numerous specific theories seeking to explain the development and maintenance of eating disorders. Among these, the one that most significantly influenced their treatment was cognitive behavioural theory

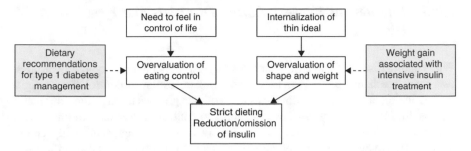

Fig. 8.3 The two pathways to eating disorders in people with type 1 diabetes, according to cognitive behavioural theory

[22, 54–56]. In brief, these theories hold that dietary restriction, a behaviour that characterizes the onset of most eating disorders, originates from two main pathways that can operate simultaneously [57]. The first occurs in individuals with a need to control various aspects of their lives (e.g. school, work, sports, other interests), when in particular circumstances they begin to shift their efforts towards the control of eating, developing the overvaluation of eating control. The second occurs in individuals who have internalized the thin ideal, and go on to develop the overvaluation of shape and weight and their control. In both cases the result is the adoption of strict dieting, which in turn reinforces the need for control over eating, shape and weight. Subsequently, other mechanisms described in Chap. 3 begin to operate and act to maintain the eating disorder psychopathology.

According to this theory, the increased prevalence of eating disorders in people with type 1 diabetes could occur because the two pathways of entry into the eating disorder "trap" are both promoted by the presence of type 1 diabetes through the following two main mechanisms (Fig. 8.3):

1. The need to feel in control is often shifted to the control of eating, particularly as regards carbohydrate intake, recommended in standard treatments for type 1 diabetes.
2. Internalization of the thin ideal can be facilitated by intensive insulin treatment, which may result in some weight gain [58].

8.2.4   Eating Disorder Psychopathology in Type 1 Diabetes

The eating disorder psychopathology of individuals with type 1 diabetes is comparable to that of those without type 1 diabetes (see Chap. 2). The only difference is that sometimes another form of body weight control is adopted through the reduction or omission of the usual insulin dose to produce conspicuous glycosuria (loss of glucose through the urine) [59].

8.2.5   Interactions Between Eating Disorders and Type 1 Diabetes

When eating disorders and type 1 diabetes coexist, they interact negatively through two main mechanisms: (i) individuals manipulate insulin to control their weight (e.g. reducing or omitting insulin doses to eliminate glucose through the urine), and (ii) insulin-induced hunger makes it difficult to control food intake. In turn, some features of eating disorders (e.g. binge-eating episodes) compromise glycaemic control. This increases the risk of diabetic coma in the short term, and specific complications of diabetes in the long term (Fig. 8.4).

8.2.6   Clinical Consequences

Eating disorders and disordered eating in individuals with type 1 diabetes are a major clinical problem because they increase the risk of diabetic ketoacidosis, hospitalization, and diabetes-related microvascular and neurological complications

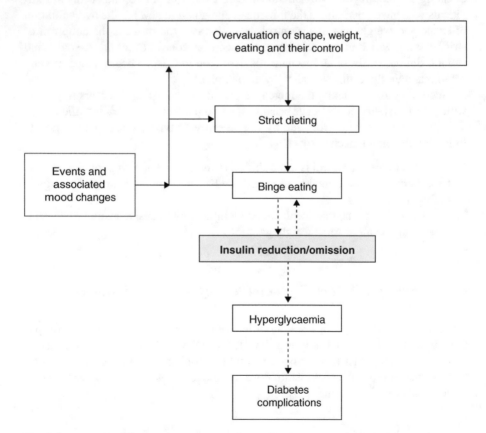

Fig. 8.4 Personalized formulation of a patient with bulimia nervosa and type 1 diabetes who omits insulin after binge-eating episodes

Table 8.4 Medical risks related to the coexistence of eating disorders with type 1 diabetes

• Higher levels of glycated haemoglobin (HbA1c)
• Higher risk of infections
• Higher rate of diabetic coma
• Higher rate of diabetes complications (retinopathy, nephropathy, neuropathy, cardiovascular complications) at an earlier age

[60, 61]. Eating disorders, including those considered subthreshold, are also associated with poor metabolic control and blood lipid abnormalities [48] that can independently increase the risk of long-term complications related to diabetes.

Eating disorders in individuals with type 1 diabetes are associated with high mortality. A Scandinavian study found that after about 10 years of follow-up, mortality rates were 2.2 (per 1000 person-years) for type 1 diabetes, 7.3 for anorexia nervosa, and 34.6 for type 1 diabetes associated with anorexia nervosa [62]. Table 8.4 summarizes the main medical risks when type 1 diabetes coexists with eating disorders.

8.2.7   Treatment

In most cases, type 1 diabetes does not hinder the psychological treatment of eating disorders, but sometimes there may be a transient deterioration in glycaemic control associated with weight regain and the introduction of avoided foods—two key CBT-E procedures for the management of eating disorders. The only CBT-E adaptation to implement is to ask the patient to report the units of insulin and daily blood sugar measurements in the Comments column of the CBT-E monitoring record (see the CBT-E manual [39]). Glycaemic index and insulin adjustment should always be monitored and managed by the patient, accompanied by the reference diabetes team, which should coordinate its intervention with the eating disorder team. In some cases, particularly in patients with anorexia nervosa and type 1 diabetes, or in those who have repeated episodes of ketoacidosis for insulin omission, hospitalization in a specialized department for the treatment of eating disorders may be indicated.

Vignette
The patient is a 16-year-old teenager with anorexia nervosa and type 1 diabetes. The diabetes arose at the age of 10, and until the age of 14 the patient scrupulously followed the indications received for the management of her insulin therapy and carb counting. At the age of 14, however, when she started high school and had a weight of 56 kg, she began to restrict her diet to lose weight and change the shape of her body, especially her legs and belly. In a few months the patient had lost 10 kg and her periods had stopped. After 6 months she started to have recurrent binge-eating episodes which she tried to compensate for by skipping her doses of insulin and fasting for one day. Such behaviour resulted in a dramatic deterioration in her

glycaemic control and an episode of ketoacidosis coma, which was treated under urgent hospitalization. After discharge, she was referred to a specialist outpatient eclectic treatment for eating disorder, which she attended for 3 months without satisfactory results. For this reason, her general practitioner referred her to us to assess whether inpatient CBT-E for eating disorder was indicated.

At the time of the assessment and preparation session, the patient weighed 36 kg (BMI 14.2) and reported following extreme and rigid dietary rules (she had eliminated carbohydrates, skipped meals, and avoided social eating), and recurrent binge-eating episodes (on average two episodes a week), which she compensated for by omitting insulin intake and fasting for an entire day. She also displayed overvaluation of shape, weight and their control; extreme fear of gaining weight; excessive and dysfunctional weight and shape checking; irritability and social withdrawal, and had stopped attending school. Her last HbA1c test result was 12% (optimal value <7%).

After having participated in four preparatory sessions, the patient agreed to be hospitalized because she had been helped to reach the conclusion that addressing weight gain and the eating disorder psychopathology would improve her glycaemic control and allow her to get back to "having a life". The patient was actively engaged in residential CBT-E-based treatment, which lasted for 3 months of hospitalization followed by 1.5 months of day-hospital. She had achieved a BMI of 19.8 at discharge. In accordance with the diabetes centre, the CBT-E therapist agreed with the patient that she would suspend carb counting (a procedure that intensified her concern about eating), and introduce a wide variety of foods to maintain a low-normal body weight, adopting flexible healthy dietary guidelines. The elimination of dietary restriction and restraint resulted in the remission of binge-eating episodes, and a marked improvement in her HbA1c (7.3% in the last week of hospitalization).

Upon completion of the programme, the patient had residual concerns about her shape, and persistent secondary amenorrhea. Thereafter, she attended 20 sessions of post-inpatient outpatient CBT-E, in which she addressed her residual body-image concerns and learned to use procedures to identify and manage early signs of reactivation of the eating disorder mindset, with a view to preventing relapse. At the post-treatment review session (40 weeks after discharge), the patient had a BMI of 20.3, regular periods, an HbA1c of 6.2% (despite no longer carb counting) and only moderate concern about the shape of her legs. She had also returned to school and spent time hanging out with her friends.

8.3   Coeliac Disease

The first report describing the association between anorexia nervosa and coeliac disease (or gluten intolerance) was published in 1966 [63]. Subsequently, other case reports on this association were reported in the early 2000s [64, 65]. However, it was only in 2017 that a longitudinal study on a large population of women was published, and found a positive and bidirectional association between coeliac disease and anorexia nervosa [66]. The coexistence of the eating disorder with coeliac

Table 8.5 General information on coeliac disease

Coeliac disease is an inherited disorder caused by sensitivity to the gliadin fraction of gluten—a protein found in wheat, but similar proteins are present in rye, barley, kamut and triticale. In a genetically susceptible individual, gluten-sensitive T cells are activated when the antigenic determinant of gluten-derived peptides is presented [67]. The inflammatory response determines the characteristic atrophy of the mucosal villi in the intestine, and consequent malabsorption of nutrients.

Like all autoimmune diseases, coeliac disease has multifactorial aetiogenesis that includes the complex interaction of genetic and environmental factors [68]. While exposure to gluten is the triggering environmental factor, genetic determinants have not yet been fully elucidated. The disease is more frequent in females (1.5–2 times more common than in males) and populations of Indo-European origin. Patients who have other diseases, such as lymphocytic colitis, Down's syndrome, type 1 diabetes and autoimmune thyroiditis (Hashimoto's disease), are at greater risk of developing coeliac disease.

Individuals with coeliac disease usually report several gastrointestinal symptoms (diarrhoea, steatorrhea, weight loss, bloating, flatulence, abdominal pain) and complications (abnormal liver function tests, iron deficiency anaemia, vitamin D and calcium deficiency, bone diseases, herpetiform dermatitis, weight loss) [69]. Affected children present growth delay, apathy and generalized hypotony, abdominal distension and muscle atrophy. However, some adult individuals do not report any symptoms [69].

Diagnosis of coeliac disease should be performed by dose screening with serological markers (e.g. total A immunoglobulins [IgA] and IgA anti-transglutaminase tissue [tTG]) and confirmed in adults via biopsy of the second portion of the duodenum. Before testing for coeliac disease, people who follow a normal diet should be advised to consume foods that contain gluten in more than one meal per day for at least 6 weeks.

The only treatment currently available for individuals with coeliac disease is the total and permanent exclusion from the diet of gluten-containing foods, which involves avoiding foods containing wheat, rye and barley. This treatment not only brings about rapid remission of symptoms associated with coeliac disease (usually clinical healing occurs in about 1–2 months from the time of gluten exclusion) but also prevents the onset of serious complications (e.g. lymphoma, bowel cancer and osteoporosis) which continuous and prolonged exposure to gluten causes in affected individuals. Ingestion of even small amounts of gluten-containing food hinders remission or causes a recurrence.

disease, especially in forms characterized by being underweight and recurrent bingeing episodes, aggravates the clinical malabsorption and increases the likelihood of developing severe complications of coeliac disease. On the other side of the coin, coeliac disease can trigger and maintain the eating disorder psychopathology in a subgroup of individuals upon the adoption of a diet that requires a total and permanent exclusion of foods containing gluten. Table 8.5 provides some general information on coeliac disease for non-medical therapists.

8.3.1 Two-Way Association between Anorexia Nervosa and Coeliac Disease

A case-controlled cohort study, carried out using the Swedish National Patient Registry, which assessed 17,959 women with coeliac disease confirmed via duodenal biopsy and 89,379 women matched by age and sex, found a positive association between coeliac disease and anorexia nervosa arising both before and after the diagnosis of coeliac disease [66]. Specifically, the study found that in women with coeliac disease diagnosed before the age of 19, the odds of a previous diagnosis of anorexia nervosa were increased 4.5-fold after having paired the data by education level, socioeconomic status and the presence of type 1 diabetes. In addition, those over 20 had an almost double risk of developing anorexia nervosa after an initial diagnosis of coeliac disease [66].

8.3.2   Mechanisms that Explain the Bidirectional Association

There are at least two factors that could explain the presence of a bidirectional association between anorexia nervosa and coeliac disease:

1. *Common genetic susceptibility*. A recent genome-wide association study identified a significant genome-wide locus for anorexia nervosa on chromosome 12, in an area previously identified as being associated with type 1 diabetes and autoimmune diseases [70]. This will hopefully prompt the study of the genetic relationship between anorexia nervosa and autoimmune gastrointestinal diseases.
2. *Surveillance bias*. Individuals with anorexia nervosa and coeliac disease are generally studied more carefully than the general population, and this can lead to more frequent diagnosis of the other condition [66].

Although coeliac disease has not yet been proven to be a risk factor for the development of eating disorders, it can be hypothesized that, in line with transdiagnostic cognitive behavioural theory [57], the presence of gastrointestinal symptoms and the need to follow a gluten-free diet may promote the onset of overvaluation of eating control and the adoption of a strict diet (Fig. 8.5)—one of the access routes to eating disorders—in individuals who have a need for control in general.

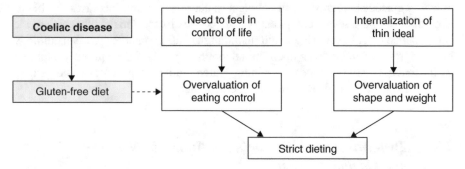

Fig. 8.5 Ways of entry to eating disorders in individuals with coeliac disease, according to cognitive behavioural theory

Table 8.6 Main signs and symptoms in common between coeliac disease and anorexia nervosa	
	• Weight loss
	• Short stature and/or thinness
	• Osteopenia/osteoporosis
	• Borborygmus
	• Meteorism
	• Abdominal distension
	• Abdominal cramps
	• Vomiting
	• Regurgitation
	• Epigastric pain
	• Heartburn
	• Asthenia
	• Iron deficiency anaemia
	• Folate and B12 deficiency anaemia

8.3.3   Attention to the Initial Diagnosis

Differential diagnosis of coeliac disease and eating disorders can be complex as many signs and symptoms are present in both disorders (Table 8.6). Usually patients present with some nonspecific abdominal symptoms (e.g. diarrhoea, abdominal bloating or pain), and the doctor's task is to identify the cause of these symptoms in order to guide the therapeutic intervention. The presence of asthenia and abdominal symptoms (in particular diarrhoea and steatorrhea) and the absence of eating disorder psychopathology (i.e. the overvaluation of shape, weight, eating and their control) are two important indications that the culprit may be coeliac disease. In this event, the first step is to prescribe the tests described above to assess for the presence of gluten intolerance. If these tests are positive, and in no other case [71], it is advisable to prescribe the patient a gluten-free diet. If, on the other hand, tests for coeliac disease are negative, and the patient reports the overvaluation of shape, weight, eating and their control, often associated with a strong fear of gaining weight, the diagnosis of an eating disorder should be considered.

8.3.4   Interaction Between Eating Disorders and Coeliac Disease

When they coexist, eating disorders and coeliac disease interact negatively with each other through numerous mechanisms (Fig. 8.6): (i) the gluten-free diet can promote an increase in eating concerns and consequently intensify dietary restriction and restraint, promoting weight loss (or hindering weight regain) and the onset of binge-eating episodes; (ii) binge-eating episodes, in which gluten-containing

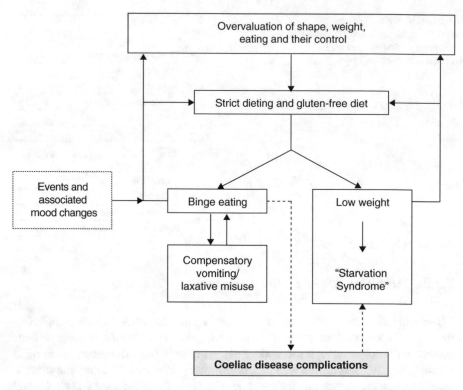

Fig. 8.6 Personalized formulation of a patient with anorexia nervosa binge-eating/purging type and coeliac disease

foods are usually ingested, keep coeliac disease active; (iii) foods containing gluten may be ingested on purpose to promote weight loss; and (iv) malnutrition and osteoporosis caused by the low weight in eating disorders can be accentuated by the malabsorption produced by coeliac disease.

8.3.5 Treatment

In most cases, the presence of coeliac disease creates an obstacle to the psychological treatment of eating disorders. Indeed, the adoption of a gluten-free diet may act to maintain eating disorder psychopathology, making it more difficult to address the high levels of dietary restraint and restriction that are key mechanisms reinforcing the eating disorder psychopathology. For this reason, the CBT-E Dietary Restriction module of the CBT-E manual [39] should be adapted to help the patient adopt a gluten-free diet and address weight regain (if indicated) at the same time. Patients should be helped to follow healthy and "flexible" dietary guidelines, inevitably excluding gluten-containing foods. Because of the nutritional risks associated with coeliac disease, a registered dietitian must be part of the eating disorder care team to monitor the patient's nutritional status [72]. Moreover, the patient should always be monitored by a doctor who is experienced in the assessment and management of malnutrition secondary to malabsorption and/or weight loss. In these cases, specific vitamin and mineral supplements may be prescribed to the patient to replenish the nutritional deficit.

Vignette

The patient is a 17-year-old teenager with anorexia nervosa and coeliac disease. She was diagnosed with the latter at the age of 14 due to the presence of asthenia, meteorism, abdominal pain and persistent diarrhoea. The patient scrupulously followed the recommendations for a gluten-free diet, and this led to remission in the asthenia and gastrointestinal symptoms. However, the change in diet was associated with a weight gain of about 5 kg over 6 months (from 53 to 58 kg), probably due to remission in the malabsorption induced by the previous intake of gluten-containing foods.

To manage her weight gain and the resulting dissatisfaction with her shape and weight, the patient began to restrict her food intake and lost 4 kg in 1 month. Dietary restriction and weight loss were accompanied by a marked increase in her concerns about eating, shape and weight. She started to count all the calories in foods, and repeatedly weigh the food she was to eat, weighing herself several times a day and repeatedly checking the shape of her stomach and legs in the mirror. These concerns, coupled with her morbid fear of gaining weight, led her to intensify her dietary restriction, even when she had reached her habitual weight of 53 kg, and in 4 months she had reached a weight of 41 kg.

From the age of 15–16, she received a specialist multidisciplinary outpatient treatment for eating disorders without any improvement, and her body weight ranged between 40 and 43 kg. At age 16, after breaking one of her dietary rules (she ate two biscuits containing gluten), she had her first binge-eating episode, which she compensated for by self-inducing vomiting. After this episode, she alternated between periods of strict dieting interrupted by recurrent episodes of objective and subjective binge-eating followed by self-induced vomiting. Her intake of gluten-containing foods during the binge-eating episodes reactivated her gastrointestinal symptoms and asthenia, which were also accentuated by her underweight and malnourished conditions.

At our assessment and preparation session, the patient weighed 37 kg (BMI 14.2) and reported following extreme and rigid dietary rules, recurrent episodes of objective (on average two episodes per week) and subjective (on average five episodes a week) binge-eating followed by self-induced vomiting, overvaluation of shape and weight, marked fear of gaining weight, and frequent weight and shape checking in the mirror. The patient also reported low mood, irritability, reduced socialization and interruption of school attendance. Recent blood tests had shown the presence of anaemia, low white blood cell count and hypokalaemia. She also reported persistent abdominal bloating and pain, recurrent episodes of diarrhoea, and secondary amenorrhea that had lasted for about 2 years.

The patient accepted the proposal to be treated via inpatient CBT-E. Actively engaged in the treatment, she developed a good therapeutic relationship and was very cooperative with the various aspects of treatment. In particular, during the day-hospital phase, she managed to maintain her weight with no binge-eating episodes or self-induced vomiting, following the dietary guidelines for the management of coeliac disease and flexibly eating non-gluten-containing food. At discharge, her impaired blood values had returned to normal, her gastrointestinal symptoms had regressed and she had a BMI of 19.5.

However, her concerns about weight and shape persisted, and after the day-hospital phase of inpatient treatment she attended the 20 planned post-inpatient CBT-E sessions. During this period she had sporadic objective binge-eating episodes triggered by events and associated mood changes, but maintained her weight, her menstrual cycle resumed, and her concerns about shape and weight were significantly reduced.

At the post-treatment review session, 20 weeks after the conclusion of post-inpatient CBT-E, the patient, at a BMI of 20, was in remission from the eating disorder, was managing her coeliac disease well by eating a gluten-free diet and was regularly attending school and spending time with friends.

8.4 Allergies

Food allergy and anaphylaxis are an increasing burden in developed countries. Prevalence is high in young children, but recent evidence indicates that they are becoming increasingly more common in teenagers and young women and, also, in developing countries [73]. However, the number of people who call themselves "allergic to food" highly overestimates the actual prevalence of food allergies [74]. This is due to misuse of the term "allergic", which is erroneously used to label side effects of drugs, toxic reactions to food, enzyme deficits (e.g. lactase or sucrase-isomaltose deficiency) and vasomotor reactions to irritants (e.g. citrus fruits or tomatoes) [75]. A further overestimation occurs when food allergies are spuriously blamed as the cause of a variety of different conditions (e.g. migraine, irritable bowel syndrome, chronic urticaria, chronic fatigue syndrome, child hyperkinetic syndrome, serum-negative arthritis, serous otitis and Crohn's disease), without the support of rigorous research [73]. This has created a widespread general opinion that food allergy may be a "medical chameleon" [75], potentially able to explain different disorders and symptoms without any specific biomarkers having been identified.

Generally, there is a notable difference between the prevalence of clinical suspicion of an adverse reaction to food (about 20%) and diagnostic confirmation (1.8%) via the double-blind placebo-controlled food challenge (considered the gold standard in the diagnosis of food allergy) [76].

Table 8.7 Some "alternative" tests for food intolerance, none of which have robust evidence to validate their use	
	• Cytotoxic test (Bryan test)
	• Provocation/neutralization sublingual or subcutaneous test
	• Bioresonance
	• Electro-acupuncture
	• Hair analysis
	• Immunological tests (immunocomplex or specific food IgG)
	• Applied kinesiology
	• Cardio-auricular reflex test
	• Pulse test
	• Vega test
	• Sarm test
	• Biostrength tests and variants
	• Natrix or FIT 184 Tests
	• BAFF (B-lymphocyte-activating factor) and PAF (platelet-activating factor) tests

8.4.1 Alternative Food Intolerance Tests

An additional and worrying source of diagnostic confusion is the phenomenon of increasingly frequent use by the population of alternative diagnostic tests [77, 78] (Table 8.7) without any scientific validity. Often recommended by healthcare personnel (e.g. pharmacist, doctor or naturopath), these tests are purported to identify, with methods other than traditional ones, the foods responsible for food allergies or food "intolerances". The latter term, which in its strictest sense indicates "any reproducible adverse reaction following the ingestion of a food or some of its components (proteins, carbohydrates, fats, preservatives), which includes toxic, metabolic and allergic reactions" [75], is increasingly also used to indicate a psychological aversion to different foods as is seen in a subgroup of patients suffering from eating disorders.

8.4.2 False Eating Intolerances and Eating Disorders

Alternative testing for food intolerance is often misused in patients with eating disorders, particularly in those suffering from functional gastrointestinal symptoms. The hypothesis behind the use of alternative tests is that the targeted elimination of certain foods to which the individual is purportedly "intolerant" produces an improvement in gastrointestinal symptoms and thus promotes the resumption of a regular diet.

However, at least one account, confirmed by numerous clinical cases that we have seen in recent years, has described cases of anorexia nervosa developing in individuals who followed diets indicated by alternative tests [79]. It reported on a series of young normal-weight women who complained of vague gastrointestinal symptoms in the absence of documented organic damage. We hypothesize that the onset of gastrointestinal symptoms in these people was triggered by stress [80] rather than intolerance to specific foods; the mediation factor between stress factors and dyspeptic symptoms could be corticotropin-releasing hormone, which, at least in patients with irritable bowel syndrome, seems to act centrally, modulating both gastric motility and gastrointestinal symptoms [81].

The risk of developing an eating disorder following the prescription of a diet which involves the elimination of several foods to reduce dyspeptic symptoms seems particularly high in adolescents and young women who have a need to feel in control in life (e.g. feeling in control in various aspects of life such as school, work, sports or other interests). Following a strict diet may trigger the shift towards eating control via two main mechanisms:

1. Eating control is experienced as a successful behaviour in a context of perceived failure in other areas of life [56].
2. Reducing caloric intake and foods such as fermentation-producing carbohydrates often results in a short-term improvement in gastrointestinal symptoms [79].

However, after a short period of improvement, gastrointestinal symptoms tend to worsen due to the combined action of various mechanisms operating simultaneously, such as paying excessive attention to abdominal sensations that are not normally noticed [56] and the negative effects of dietary restriction and weight loss on gastric emptying [80]. These factors, associated with the overvaluation of eating control and morbid fear that the introduction of "intolerable" foods may exacerbate gastrointestinal symptoms, thereby maintain and intensify the eating disorder psychopathology (Fig. 8.7).

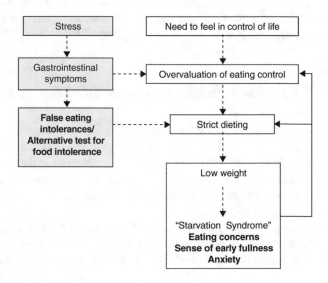

Fig. 8.7 Interaction between misdiagnosis of food intolerance and maintenance of eating-disorder psychopathology

Diets that require the elimination of several foods, such as those "indicated" by alternative food intolerance tests, also seem to be a trigger and maintenance mechanism for binge-eating episodes [22]. Attempting to limit food intake, regardless of whether or not it produces an energy deficit, requires the adoption of extreme and rigid dietary rules. The (almost inevitable) breaking of these rules is often interpreted as evidence of lack of self-control, resulting in temporary abandonment of eating control and the intake of a large amount of food. In turn, the binge-eating episode intensifies concerns about eating, shape, weight and their control, which encourages further dietary restriction, resulting in an increased risk of a new binge-eating episode.

8.4.3 Treatment

In the event that a patient reports food intolerance, they will need referring to a qualified allergist, who will be able to educate the patient whether or not this is, in fact, the case. An evidence-based psychological treatment such as CBT-E [39, 82] may then be useful in encouraging such patients to gradually re-introduce avoided foods and restore weight (if indicated), while helping them develop a more articulated self-evaluation scheme not predominantly based on the control of eating, shape and weight.

Vignette

The patient is a young woman of 19 years of age who, after failing the entrance test for medical school, began to manifest recurrent dyspeptic symptoms, in particular bloating and pain in the upper abdomen and postprandial heaviness. A gastroenterologist she consulted prescribed a series of exams (i.e. helicobacter pylori screening, oesophagogastroduodenoscopy, gastric emptying study), which revealed no gastrointestinal abnormalities. The patient then consulted a nutritionist who, after performing a non-scientific food intolerance test (i.e. Vega test), advised her to cut out numerous foods, including bread, pasta, wheat, milk and dairy products. The patient scrupulously adhered to the exclusion diet and experienced an immediate improvement in the dyspeptic symptoms. She was thereby convinced that she was truly intolerant to these foods, and, upon the recurrence of her dyspeptic symptom a few weeks later, decided to cut out still more foods (i.e. meat, fish, legumes, cabbage, broccoli and mushrooms) from her diet. She began to lose weight rapidly, and her periods stopped.

At our assessment and preparation session, the patient weighed 38 kg (her usual weight was 55 kg), and reported following a strict low-calorie diet characterized by the daily intake of only a small amount of white rice, one piece of fruit, and sometimes a small portion of chicken breast. The patient did not report a fear of gaining weight—indeed she was very concerned about her low weight—but avoided eating numerous foods for fear of accentuating her dyspeptic symptoms. However, despite the strict diet, she still experienced frequent pains in her upper abdomen, a sense of early fullness, and long and difficult digestion. She also reported frequent mood swings, irritability, social withdrawal and difficulty concentrating on her studies. She described herself as having been a cheerful person before her dramatic weight loss, with many interest and friendships.

After recording the patient's history, the CBT-E therapist informed her that the dyspeptic symptoms might have been the result of a stressful situation producing an alteration in gastrointestinal function. He explained that the elimination of certain food was maintaining and accentuating the problem because, after an initial improvement in symptoms due to the dietary restriction that "rested" her stomach, the dietary restriction and weight loss produced a gastric emptying slowdown; as a consequence, she experienced the feeling of premature fullness and her abdominal bloating and pain worsened. Her avoidance of other foods as a consequence led to further deterioration in nutritional status and dyspeptic symptoms. To help the patient accept this idea, the therapist asked the patient whether she would agree to be assessed by an allergist—an expert in food allergies and intolerance. She consented, and allergy testing excluded the presence of any food allergy or intolerance.

For this reason, the patient decided with some reluctance to start outpatient CBT-E, and after 3 weeks of Step One, the regular eating procedure led to a reduction in her sense of early fullness and abdominal bloating and pain. This motivated the patient to undertake CBT-E Step Two, in which she accepted weight regain and the gradual introduction of avoided foods. In addition, the treatment addressed her overvaluation of eating control and, after normalization of body weight, setbacks and mindset to manage early signs of relapse. Finally, Step CBT-E Three introduced procedures to conclude the treatment well, address residual problems and prevent relapse. At the post-treatment review session, 20 weeks after the conclusion of CBT-E, the patient weighed 56 kg, had a regular menstrual cycle and reported no longer experiencing digestive problems.

8.5   Other Coexisting Medical Problems

In a small minority of patients, other general medical conditions such as inflammatory bowel disease (i.e. Crohn's disease or ulcerative colitis) or irritable bowel syndrome can coexist with the eating disorder psychopathology. In these cases, the therapist should evaluate the following characteristics: (i) the interaction between the eating disorder and the general medical disease, (ii) the effect of the eating disorder on the general medical disease, (iii) the effect of treatment on the general medical disease and (iv) any possible adaptations, always slight, to be made to way in which the eating disorder is treated.

References

1. Fairburn CG, Cooper Z, Waller D. Complex cases and comorbidity. In: Fairburn CG, editor. Cognitive behavior therapy and eating disorders. New York: Guilford Press; 2008.
2. Bray GA, Kim KK, Wilding JPH. Obesity: a chronic relapsing progressive disease process. A position statement of the world obesity federation. Obes Rev. 2017;18(7):715–23. https://doi.org/10.1111/obr.12551.
3. World Health Organization. Obesity and overweight; 2020. Available from: https://www.who.int/en/news-room/fact-sheets/detail/obesity-and-overweight.
4. Rose KM, Newman B, Mayer-Davis EJ, Selby JV. Genetic and behavioral determinants of waist-hip ratio and waist circumference in women twins. Obes Res. 1998;6(6):383–92. https://doi.org/10.1002/j.1550-8528.1998.tb00369.x.
5. Field AE, Sonneville KR, Micali N, Crosby RD, Swanson SA, Laird NM, et al. Prospective association of common eating disorders and adverse outcomes. Pediatrics. 2012;130(2):e289–95. https://doi.org/10.1542/peds.2011-3663.
6. Ness-Abramof R, Apovian CM. Drug-induced weight gain. Drugs Today (Barc). 2005;41(8):547–55. https://doi.org/10.1358/dot.2005.41.8.893630.
7. Kolotkin RL, Andersen JR. A systematic review of reviews: exploring the relationship between obesity, weight loss and health-related quality of life. Clin Obes. 2017;7(5):273–89. https://doi.org/10.1111/cob.12203.
8. Visser M, Langlois J, Guralnik JM, Cauley JA, Kronmal RA, Robbins J, et al. High body fatness, but not low fat-free mass, predicts disability in older men and women: the cardiovascular health study. Am J Clin Nutr. 1998;68(3):584–90. https://doi.org/10.1093/ajcn/68.3.584.
9. Global BMIMC, Di Angelantonio E, Bhupathiraju Sh N, Wormser D, Gao P, Kaptoge S, et al. Body-mass index and all-cause mortality: individual-participant-data meta-analysis of 239 prospective studies in four continents. Lancet. 2016;388(10046):776–86. https://doi.org/10.1016/s0140-6736(16)30175-1.
10. Pearl RL, Puhl RM. Weight bias internalization and health: a systematic review. Obes Rev. 2018;19(8):1141–63. https://doi.org/10.1111/obr.12701.
11. Allison KC, Crow SJ, Reeves RR, West DS, Foreyt JP, Dilillo VG, et al. Binge eating disorder and night eating syndrome in adults with type 2 diabetes. Obesity (Silver Spring, Md). 2007;15(5):1287–93. https://doi.org/10.1038/oby.2007.150.
12. Gorin AA, Niemeier HM, Hogan P, Coday M, Davis C, DiLillo VG, et al. Binge eating and weight loss outcomes in overweight and obese individuals with type 2 diabetes: results from the look AHEAD trial. Arch Gen Psychiatry. 2008;65(12):1447–55. https://doi.org/10.1001/archpsyc.65.12.1447.
13. Ricca V, Mannucci E, Moretti S, Di Bernardo M, Zucchi T, Cabras PL, et al. Screening for binge eating disorder in obese outpatients. Compr Psychiatry. 2000;41(2):111–5. https://doi.org/10.1016/s0010-440x(00)90143-3.
14. Fairburn CG, Welch SL, Doll HA, Davies BA, O'Connor ME. Risk factors for bulimia nervosa. A community-based case-control study. Arch Gen Psychiatry. 1997;54(6):509–17. https://doi.org/10.1001/archpsyc.1997.01830180015003.
15. Fairburn CG, Doll HA, Welch SL, Hay PJ, Davies BA, O'Connor ME. Risk factors for binge eating disorder: a community-based, case-control study. Arch Gen Psychiatry. 1998;55(5):425–32. https://doi.org/10.1001/archpsyc.55.5.425.
16. Hilbert A, Pike KM, Goldschmidt AB, Wilfley DE, Fairburn CG, Dohm FA, et al. Risk factors across the eating disorders. Psychiatry Res. 2014;220(1–2):500–6. https://doi.org/10.1016/j.psychres.2014.05.054.
17. Allen KL, Schmidt U. Risck factors for eating disorders. In: Brownell KD, Walsh BT, editors. Eating disorders and obesity. New York: Guilford Press; 2017. p. 254–9.
18. Cooper Z, Calugi S, Dalle Grave R. Controlling binge eating and weight: a treatment for binge eating disorder worth researching? Eat Weight Disord. 2019. https://doi.org/10.1007/s40519-019-00734-4.

19. Hudson JI, Lalonde JK, Coit CE, Tsuang MT, McElroy SL, Crow SJ, et al. Longitudinal study of the diagnosis of components of the metabolic syndrome in individuals with binge-eating disorder. Am J Clin Nutr. 2010;91(6):1568–73. https://doi.org/10.3945/ajcn.2010.29203.
20. Mitchell JE, King WC, Pories W, Wolfe B, Flum DR, Spaniolas K, et al. Binge eating disorder and medical comorbidities in bariatric surgery candidates. Int J Eat Disord. 2015;48(5):471–6. https://doi.org/10.1002/eat.22389.
21. Bulik CM, Reichborn-Kjennerud T. Medical morbidity in binge eating disorder. Int J Eat Disord. 2003;34(Suppl):S39–46. https://doi.org/10.1002/eat.10204.
22. Fairburn CG, Cooper Z, Shafran R. Cognitive behaviour therapy for eating disorders: a "transdiagnostic" theory and treatment. Behav Res Ther. 2003;41(5):509–28. https://doi.org/10.1016/s0005-7967(02)00088-8.
23. Dalle Grave R, Sartirana M, El Ghoch M, Calugi S. Adapting CBT-OB for binge-eating disorder. Treating obesity with personalized cognitive behavioral therapy. Cham: Springer; 2018. p. 195–210.
24. Grilo CM. Psychological and behavioral treatments for binge-eating disorder. J Clin Psychiatry. 2017;78(Suppl 1):20–4. https://doi.org/10.4088/JCP.sh16003su1c.04.
25. Wilson GT. Treatment of binge eating disorder. Psychiatr Clin North Am. 2011;34(4):773–83. https://doi.org/10.1016/j.psc.2011.08.011.
26. Hilbert A, Petroff D, Herpertz S, Pietrowsky R, Tuschen-Caffier B, Vocks S, et al. Meta-analysis of the efficacy of psychological and medical treatments for binge-eating disorder. J Consult Clin Psychol. 2019;87(1):91–105. https://doi.org/10.1037/ccp0000358.
27. Grilo CM, Masheb RM, Salant SL. Cognitive behavioral therapy guided self-help and orlistat for the treatment of binge eating disorder: a randomized, double-blind, placebo-controlled trial. Biol Psychiatry. 2005;57(10):1193–201. https://doi.org/10.1016/j.biopsych.2005.03.001.
28. Masheb RM, Grilo CM, Rolls BJ. A randomized controlled trial for obesity and binge eating disorder: low-energy-density dietary counseling and cognitive-behavioral therapy. Behav Res Ther. 2011;49(12):821–9. https://doi.org/10.1016/j.brat.2011.09.006.
29. Blanchet C, Mathieu M, St-Laurent A, Fecteau S, St-Amour N, Drapeau V. A systematic review of physical activity interventions in individuals with binge eating disorders. Curr Obes Rep. 2018;7(1):76–88. https://doi.org/10.1007/s13679-018-0295-x.
30. Devlin MJ. Binge eating disorder. In: Brownell KD, Walsh BT, editors. Eating disorders and obesity. New York: Guilford Press; 2017. p. 192–7.
31. Linardon J, Wade TD, de la Piedad GX, Brennan L. The efficacy of cognitive-behavioral therapy for eating disorders: a systematic review and meta-analysis. J Consult Clin Psychol. 2017;85(11):1080–94. https://doi.org/10.1037/ccp0000245.
32. Cooper Z, Doll HA, Hawker DM, Byrne S, Bonner G, Eeley E, et al. Testing a new cognitive behavioural treatment for obesity: a randomized controlled trial with three-year follow-up. Behav Res Ther. 2010;48(8):706–13. https://doi.org/10.1016/j.brat.2010.03.008.
33. Dalle Grave R, Calugi S, Bosco G, Valerio L, Valenti C, El Ghoch M, et al. Personalized group cognitive behavioural therapy for obesity: a longitudinal study in a real-world clinical setting. Eat Weight Disord. 2018; https://doi.org/10.1007/s40519-018-0593-z.
34. Hagan KE, Forbush KT, Chen PY. Is dietary restraint a unitary or multi-faceted construct? Psychol Assess. 2017;29(10):1249–60. https://doi.org/10.1037/pas0000429.
35. Blomquist KK, Grilo CM. Predictive significance of changes in dietary restraint in obese patients with binge eating disorder during treatment. Int J Eat Disord. 2011;44(6):515–23. https://doi.org/10.1002/eat.20849.
36. Szmukler GI. Anorexia nervosa and bulimia in diabetics. J Psychosom Res. 1984;28(5):365–9. https://doi.org/10.1016/0022-3999(84)90067-9.
37. Young V, Eiser C, Johnson B, Brierley S, Epton T, Elliott J, et al. Eating problems in adolescents with type 1 diabetes: a systematic review with meta-analysis. Diabet Med. 2013;30(2):189–98. https://doi.org/10.1111/j.1464-5491.2012.03771.x.

38. Pinhas-Hamiel O, Hamiel U, Levy-Shraga Y. Eating disorders in adolescents with type 1 diabetes: challenges in diagnosis and treatment. World J Diabetes. 2015;6(3):517–26. https://doi.org/10.4239/wjd.v6.i3.517.

39. Dalle Grave R, Calugi S. Cognitive behavior therapy for adolescents with eating disorders. New York: Guilford Press; 2020.

40. World Health Organization. Diabetes: key facts; 2020. Available from: https://www.who.int/en/news-room/fact-sheets/detail/diabetes.

41. Torpy JM, Lynm C, Glass RM. Type 1 diabetes. JAMA. 2007;298(12):1472. https://doi.org/10.1001/jama.298.12.1472.

42. National Institute of Diabetes & Digestive & Kidney Diseases. Symptoms & causes of diabetes. Available from: https://www.niddk.nih.gov/health-information/diabetes/overview/symptoms-causes?dkrd=hiscr0005.

43. Chiang JL, Kirkman MS, Laffel LM, Peters AL. Type 1 diabetes through the life span: a position statement of the American Diabetes Association. Diabetes Care. 2014;37(7):2034–54. https://doi.org/10.2337/dc14-1140.

44. Diseases NIoDDK. Diabetes diet, eating, & physical activity. Available from: https://www.niddk.nih.gov/health-information/diabetes/overview/diet-eating-physical-activity.

45. Markowitz JT, Butler DA, Volkening LK, Antisdel JE, Anderson BJ, Laffel LM. Brief screening tool for disordered eating in diabetes: internal consistency and external validity in a contemporary sample of pediatric patients with type 1 diabetes. Diabetes Care. 2010;33(3):495–500. https://doi.org/10.2337/dc09-1890.

46. Mannucci E, Rotella F, Ricca V, Moretti S, Placidi GF, Rotella CM. Eating disorders in patients with type 1 diabetes: a meta-analysis. J Endocrinol Investig. 2005;28(5):417–9. https://doi.org/10.1007/bf03347221.

47. Yan L. 'Diabulimia' a growing problem among diabetic girls. Nephrol News Issues. 2007;21(11):36, 8.

48. Wisting L, Froisland DH, Skrivarhaug T, Dahl-Jorgensen K, Ro O. Disturbed eating behavior and omission of insulin in adolescents receiving intensified insulin treatment: a nationwide population-based study. Diabetes Care. 2013;36(11):3382–7. https://doi.org/10.2337/dc13-0431.

49. Cherubini V, Skrami E, Iannilli A, Cesaretti A, Paparusso AM, Alessandrelli MC, et al. Disordered eating behaviors in adolescents with type 1 diabetes: a cross-sectional population-based study in Italy. Int J Eat Disord. 2018; https://doi.org/10.1002/eat.22889.

50. American Psychiatric Association. Diagnostic and statistical manual of mental disorders, (DSM-5). Arlington: American Psychiatric Publishing; 2013.

51. Watson HJ, Yilmaz Z, Thornton LM, Hübel C, Coleman JRI, Gaspar HA, et al. Genome-wide association study identifies eight risk loci and implicates metabo-psychiatric origins for anorexia nervosa. Nat Genet. 2019; https://doi.org/10.1038/s41588-019-0439-2.

52. de Groot M, Anderson R, Freedland KE, Clouse RE, Lustman PJ. Association of depression and diabetes complications: a meta-analysis. Psychosom Med. 2001;63(4):619–30. https://doi.org/10.1097/00006842-200107000-00015.

53. Domargård A, Särnblad S, Kroon M, Karlsson I, Skeppner G, Aman J. Increased prevalence of overweight in adolescent girls with type 1 diabetes mellitus. Acta Paediatr. 1999;88(11):1223–8. https://doi.org/10.1080/080352599750030329.

54. Garner DM, Bemis KM. A cognitive-behavioral approach to anorexia nervosa. Cognit Ther Res. 1982;6(2):123–50. https://doi.org/10.1007/bf01183887.

55. Slade P. Towards a functional analysis of anorexia nervosa and bulimia nervosa. Br J Clin Psychol. 1982;21(3):167–79. https://doi.org/10.1111/j.2044-8260.1982.tb00549.x.

56. Fairburn CG, Shafran R, Cooper Z. A cognitive behavioural theory of anorexia nervosa. Behav Res Ther. 1999;37(1):1–13. https://doi.org/10.1016/s0005-7967(98)00102-8.

57. Fairburn CG, Harrison PJ. Eating disorders. Lancet. 2003;361(9355):407–16. https://doi.org/10.1016/s0140-6736(03)12378-1.

58. Larger E. Weight gain and insulin treatment. Diabetes Metab. 2005;31(4 Pt 2):4s51–4s6. https://doi.org/10.1016/s1262-3636(05)88268-0.
59. Goebel-Fabbri A. Prevention and recovery from eating disorders in type 1 diabetes: injecting hope. New York, NY: Routledge; 2017.
60. Rydall AC, Rodin GM, Olmsted MP, Devenyi RG, Daneman D. Disordered eating behavior and microvascular complications in young women with insulin-dependent diabetes mellitus. N Engl J Med. 1997;336(26):1849–54. https://doi.org/10.1056/nejm199706263362601.
61. Peveler RC, Bryden KS, Neil HA, Fairburn CG, Mayou RA, Dunger DB, et al. The relationship of disordered eating habits and attitudes to clinical outcomes in young adult females with type 1 diabetes. Diabetes Care. 2005;28(1):84–8. https://doi.org/10.2337/diacare.28.1.84.
62. Nielsen S, Emborg C, Molbak AG. Mortality in concurrent type 1 diabetes and anorexia nervosa. Diabetes Care. 2002;25(2):309–12. https://doi.org/10.2337/diacare.25.2.309.
63. Ferrara A, Fontana VJ. Celiac disease and anorexia nervosa. N Y State J Med. 1966;66(8):1000–5.
64. Yucel B, Ozbey N, Demir K, Polat A, Yager J. Eating disorders and celiac disease: a case report. Int J Eat Disord. 2006;39(6):530–2. https://doi.org/10.1002/eat.20294.
65. Ricca V, Mannucci E, Calabro A, Bernardo MD, Cabras PL, Rotella CM. Anorexia nervosa and celiac disease: two case reports. Int J Eat Disord. 2000;27(1):119–22. https://doi.org/10.1002/(sici)1098-108x(200001)27:1<119::aid-eat16>3.0.co;2-r.
66. Marild K, Stordal K, Bulik CM, Rewers M, Ekbom A, Liu E, et al. Celiac disease and anorexia nervosa: a nationwide study. Pediatrics. 2017;139(5) https://doi.org/10.1542/peds.2016-4367.
67. Ruiz AR. Malattia celiaca—Disturbi gastrointestinali. Manuali MSD Edizione Professionisti. 2018;
68. Wolters VM, Wijmenga C. Genetic background of celiac disease and its clinical implications. Am J Gastroenterol. 2008;103(1):190–5. https://doi.org/10.1111/j.1572-0241.2007.01471.x.
69. Rubio-Tapia A, Hill ID, Kelly CP, Calderwood AH, Murray JA. American College of G. ACG clinical guidelines: diagnosis and management of celiac disease. Am J Gastroenterol. 2013;108(5):656–76; quiz 77. https://doi.org/10.1038/ajg.2013.79.
70. Duncan L, Yilmaz Z, Gaspar H, Walters R, Goldstein J, Anttila V, et al. Significant locus and metabolic genetic correlations revealed in genome-wide association study of anorexia nervosa. Am J Psychiatry. 2017;174(9):850–8. https://doi.org/10.1176/appi.ajp.2017.16121402.
71. Gaesser GA, Angadi SS. Gluten-free diet: imprudent dietary advice for the general population? J Acad Nutr Diet. 2012;112(9):1330–3. https://doi.org/10.1016/j.jand.2012.06.009.
72. Kupper C. Dietary guidelines and implementation for celiac disease. Gastroenterology. 2005;128(4 Suppl 1):S121–7. https://doi.org/10.1053/j.gastro.2005.02.024.
73. Tang ML, Mullins RJ. Food allergy: is prevalence increasing? Intern Med J. 2017;47(3):256–61. https://doi.org/10.1111/imj.13362.
74. Woods RK, Stoney RM, Raven J, Walters EH, Abramson M, Thien FC. Reported adverse food reactions overestimate true food allergy in the community. Eur J Clin Nutr. 2002;56(1):31–6. https://doi.org/10.1038/sj.ejcn.1601306.
75. Senna G, Passalacqua G, Lombardi C, Antonicelli L, Dalle Grave R. Diagnostica delle allergopatie e test "alternativi". MD Medicina Doctor. 2008;31:28–35.
76. Bindslev-Jensen C, Ballmer-Weber BK, Bengtsson U, Blanco C, Ebner C, Hourihane J, et al. Standardization of food challenges in patients with immediate reactions to foods—position paper from the European academy of Allergology and clinical immunology. Allergy. 2004;59(7):690–7. https://doi.org/10.1111/j.1398-9995.2004.00466.x.
77. Senna G, Gani F, Leo G, Schiappoli M. Alternative tests in the diagnosis of food allergies. Recenti Prog Med. 2002;93(5):327–34.
78. Senna G, Bonadonna P, Schiappoli M, Leo G, Lombardi C, Passalacqua G. Pattern of use and diagnostic value of complementary/alternative tests for adverse reactions to food. Allergy. 2005;60(9):1216–7. https://doi.org/10.1111/j.1398-9995.2005.00875.x.

79. Dalle Grave R, Calugi S, Marchesini G. Underweight eating disorder without over-evaluation of shape and weight: atypical anorexia nervosa? Int J Eat Disord. 2008;41(8):705–12. https://doi.org/10.1002/eat.20555.

80. Benini L, Todesco T, Dalle Grave R, Deiorio F, Salandini L, Vantini I. Gastric emptying in patients with restricting and binge/purging subtypes of anorexia nervosa. Am J Gastroenterol. 2004;99(8):1448–54. https://doi.org/10.1111/j.1572-0241.2004.30246.x.

81. Fukudo S, Nomura T, Hongo M. Impact of corticotropin-releasing hormone on gastrointestinal motility and adrenocorticotropic hormone in normal controls and patients with irritable bowel syndrome. Gut. 1998;42(6):845–9. https://doi.org/10.1136/gut.42.6.845.

82. Fairburn CG. Cognitive behavior therapy and eating disorders. New York: Guilford Press; 2008.

Chapter 9
Severe and Enduring Anorexia Nervosa

In some patients, anorexia nervosa is of brief duration and remits without treatment or after a short-term intervention, but in others it tends to persist, necessitating long and complex specialized treatments. Unfortunately, about 20% of individuals with anorexia nervosa do not improve with any of the treatments available to date, and go on to develop a lifelong condition, often associated with severe physical and psychosocial impairment. Unfortunately, there is no consensus among clinicians and researchers on how to define and treat these cases.

9.1 Labels and Definitions Used for Patients with Enduring Anorexia Nervosa

Several labels have been used to characterize patients with enduring forms of anorexia nervosa (Table 9.1) [1]. Definitions can help communication between professionals and may also stigmatize patients suffering from mental illness.

Table 9.1 Common labels used for the severe and enduring form of anorexia nervosa

• Chronic
• Refractory
• Recalcitrant
• Treatment-resistant
• Treatment-refractory
• Critical
• Severe
• Prolonged
• Long-standing
• Enduring
• Severe and enduring

© The Author(s), under exclusive license to Springer Nature Switzerland AG 2021
R. Dalle Grave et al., *Complex Cases and Comorbidity in Eating Disorders*,
https://doi.org/10.1007/978-3-030-69341-1_9

Furthermore, the impact of the words used in the definitions can influence how patients and their families experience the disease—language sends powerful messages on identity and prognosis of diseases or disorders.

"Chronic" anorexia nervosa is still the label most commonly applied to enduring forms of anorexia nervosa. However, no unmodifiable biomarkers for anorexia nervosa have been discovered, and some patients fully recover after several years of the disorder—two features that should prevent the use of the term "chronic" [2]. Moreover, describing an illness as "chronic", "treatment-resistant", "refractory" or "recalcitrant" may have a profound impact on the management of anorexia nervosa and how patients experience their disorder. Hence, other terms that are less focused on the patients' possibility of recovery, instead labelling the severity (e.g., severe) and duration (e.g., enduring or long-standing), may be more appropriate. For this reason, we discuss "severe and enduring" anorexia nervosa in this chapter.

The aim of severity specifiers for anorexia nervosa is to help provide an index of both the intensity of the psychopathological features of the disorder and the associated level of functional impairment. Furthermore, severity specifiers should enable clinicians to recommend more appropriate treatments for anorexia nervosa based on the severity of its presentation. According to the DSM-5 [3], the level of anorexia nervosa severity is not based on the duration of the disorder, but on current BMI for adults or corresponding BMI-for-age percentiles for children. However, BMI has been revealed as a poor predictor of long-term outcomes and mortality in anorexia nervosa [4], and the DSM-5 BMI-based severity specifiers for anorexia nervosa seem to have limited clinical utility in predicting treatment outcome [5]. Hence, there is the need to identify alternative clinical variables able to provide more robust prognostic indicators of treatment response in anorexia nervosa.

One potential severity specifier for anorexia nervosa is the duration of the disorder. However, although the most common duration criterion for enduring anorexia nervosa is a presentation of the disorder for at least 7 years [1], it ranges from 3–10 years [6], and data on the prognostic effect of disorder duration are inconsistent [6]. While some studies have found an association between anorexia nervosa duration and poor response [7, 8], others, using CBT-E, including a study conducted by our team, found that duration of illness had no discernible effect on treatment response [9, 10]. Furthermore, a long-term follow-up study (which spanned over 30 years) demonstrated that a progressively larger proportion of patients with anorexia nervosa achieve remission from the disorder over the long term [11]. It has been observed in another study that about 30% of patients with anorexia nervosa achieve remission in the first decade of the disorder, and about another 30% in the second decade [12].

Patients with anorexia nervosa are also categorized on the basis of previous treatment failures, but this is also difficult to define [6]. Should we consider any eating disorder treatment, whether psychiatric, psychological or clinical, previous hospitalizations, or only evidence-based treatment? Similarly, a patient's age is a problematic means of classifying patients [6]. For example, a young woman, 21 years of age, could be considered a patient with "chronic" anorexia nervosa if the age of onset of the disorder was 13; such a categorization may unduly influence the treatment strategy, prematurely indicating the harm reduction approach that is increasingly seen as the best way to manage patients with enduring anorexia nervosa. In short, both of these severity specifiers are based on the assumption that the patient has not achieved remission, and it is therefore unlikely to respond to treatment in the future. However, the data from long-term follow-up outcome studies challenge the clinical belief that patients with enduring anorexia nervosa have no hope of recovery. Moreover, the outcomes in studies assessing the effects of CBT-E suggest that many patients with enduring anorexia nervosa can achieve remission with a short-term treatment [6].

Recently Hay and Touyz suggested classification criteria for severe and enduring anorexia nervosa, taking into account both duration, treatment failure and the persistent and severe nature of the eating disorder psychopathology (i.e., a persistent state of dietary restriction, underweight, and overvaluation of shape and weight with functional impairment). The duration criterion (i.e., > 3 years) [13] is similar to that used for psychosis [14], and unsuccessful treatment is defined as exposure to at least two appropriately delivered evidence-based treatments. However, these criteria are not yet supported by empirical data concerning either the severity of the eating disorder or the predicted response to future treatments.

9.2 Which Treatment Is Indicated for Patients with Severe and Enduring Anorexia Nervosa?

The inconsistent results for all variables proposed as treatment outcome predictors mean that to date we have no good definition of severe and enduring anorexia nervosa that may reliably inform clinical practice. However, we cannot ignore the fact that there is a large group of patients with severe and enduring anorexia nervosa who are not receiving adequate treatment for their disorder. Some of these patients are refused treatment, in particular in countries that rely heavily on private health insurance (e.g., United States) [6], or are managed via strategies or procedures developed for young patients, or methods designed to coerce or force them to increase their weight (e.g., refeeding). As these methods fail to address the underlying eating disorder pathology, it will come as no surprise that they are often followed by "weight relapse" and a revolving door pattern of admission and discharge [2].

Unfortunately, there are no easy solutions for the proper treatment of these patients, and alongside the more traditional treatments designed to address the eating disorder psychopathology and weight regain, there is a new focus on management strategies designed to enhance the quality of life and reduce harm rather than promote weight gain and symptom reduction.

9.2.1 Management Strategies Designed to Enhance the Quality of Life and Reduce Harm

In the 1980s, clinicians began to recognize the difficulties in managing patients with severe and enduring anorexia nervosa, and to suggest specific recommendations for this subgroup of patients [15–18]. The strategies and procedures proposed for their management diverged from the traditional approach to eating disorder treatment, and were largely based on personal clinical experience and some theoretical considerations. They have recently been summarized by Wonderlich et al. as follows [6]:

- Clinicians should tolerate and manage extreme ambivalence or resistance to weight regain in patients with severe and enduring anorexia nervosa, and not focus their efforts primarily on weight gain.
- Patients with severe and enduring anorexia nervosa should best be treated by a comprehensive, multidisciplinary team able to provide different levels of care. Some clinicians recommended a treatment based on psychiatric rehabilitation, similar to that used for schizophrenia.
- Rather than emphasizing meal planning or significant increases in food consumption, along with weight gain it is better to pursue alternative goals, such as improving quality of life and social adjustment.
- Clinicians should consider the judicious use of legal interventions in some patients with severe and enduring anorexia nervosa.
- The involvement of family members may aid the implementation of a range of interventions, from collecting information on previous treatments to psychoeducation about eating disorders and providing general support.

However, following these general recommendations would result in a situation in which patients with severe and enduring anorexia nervosa continued to receive a broad range of poorly defined interventions with nebulous intensity, duration and goals, and a lack of integration across different levels of care [19]. This was the case even as late as 2012, when two structured treatments for severe and enduring anorexia nervosa were being designed and assessed in a randomized controlled trial. That trial was conducted in 63 patients with anorexia nervosa of at least 7 years duration with moderately severe low weight (mean BMI 16.2) [20], half of whom received specialist supportive clinical management and half CBT for severe and enduring anorexia nervosa. Both of these approaches were administered with a view to enhancing the quality of life and reducing harm, rather than increasing weight and ameliorating symptoms, and both were delivered in 30 sessions over 8 months. Both treatments are described in detail in a dedicated manual [21], and produced comparable improvements in quality of life along with a very modest weight gain (about 0.5 BMI increase). Symptoms were also improved, with CBT patients scoring slightly better in terms of social adjustment at end of treatment and eating disorder psychopathology at 12 months, and outcomes were stable at 12-month follow-up. Moreover, the rate of attrition in both programmes was only around 15%. Although these findings are promising in that they show that some patients with severe and enduring anorexia nervosa can obtain benefit from treatments designed to enhance quality of life and harm reduction, this does nothing to alleviate concerns related to the maintenance of persistent low body weight. Indeed, remaining malnourished will inevitably lead to long-term medical and psychosocial complications that, in turn, deteriorate the quality of life even further.

9.2.2   Treatments Designed to Address the Eating Disorder Psychopathology and Weight Regain

Unlike the management strategies aimed at quality-of-life enhancement and harm reduction in patients with anorexia nervosa described in the previous section, CBT-E is designed to address both weight gain and the eating disorder psychopathology, giving patients an opportunity to recover from their eating disorder. As described in Chap. 3, CBT-E is an evidence-based treatment recommended for all the eating disorder diagnostic categories in both adults and adolescents [22–24]. The aims of the treatment are as follows (see also Chap. 3) [23]:

• To engage patients in the treatment and involve them actively in the process of change
• To remove the eating disorder psychopathology, i.e., dietary restraint and restriction (and low weight if present), extreme weight-control behaviours, and preoccupation with shape, weight, and eating
• To correct the mechanisms maintaining the eating disorder psychopathology
• To ensure lasting change

Three studies, two carried out by our team, have assessed the effectiveness of CBT-E in patients with severe and enduring anorexia nervosa. The first evaluated the effects of inpatient CBT-E in 37 consecutively admitted female patients with long-standing anorexia nervosa ($\geq$10 years) and 58 with shorter duration of the disorder [25]. Individuals with long-standing anorexia nervosa had higher age, baseline BMI, higher frequency of self-induced vomiting and laxative and diuretic misuse, but, importantly, no different personality traits at baseline. Two operational outcome categories were used: (i) good BMI outcome (i.e., the achievement of BMI $\geq$18.5 kg, and (ii) full response (i.e., global Eating Disorder Examination [EDE] interview score below one standard deviation above the community mean, i.e., <1.74). Interestingly, there was no significant difference in drop-out rate between patients with long-standing and shorter-duration anorexia nervosa, and in fact a slightly higher percentage of the former completed the programme (32.4% versus 20.7%, respectively). Although the sample size was small, this seems to suggest that CBT-E is at least as well received in patients with enduring eating disorder as it is by those with the same disorder of more recent onset. Equally, if not more, encouraging was the finding that good BMI outcome was achieved by all completers with long-standing anorexia nervosa as compared to 78.3% of the short duration group. Moreover, no differences were found between enduring and recent-onset groups in terms of full response rates (62.5% vs. 48.9%, respectively) [25].

The second study we undertook evaluated the short- and long-term outcomes of CBT-E in 32 consecutive patients with anorexia nervosa defined as severe and enduring (i.e., duration of illness >7 years), and 34 with anorexia nervosa of more recent onset [9]. Both groups had a drop-out rate of around 15%, and both sets of completers displayed similarly large increases in BMI, as well as improvements in eating disorder and general psychopathology scores, with minimal deterioration after discharge (Fig. 9.1). As above, patients with severe and enduring anorexia

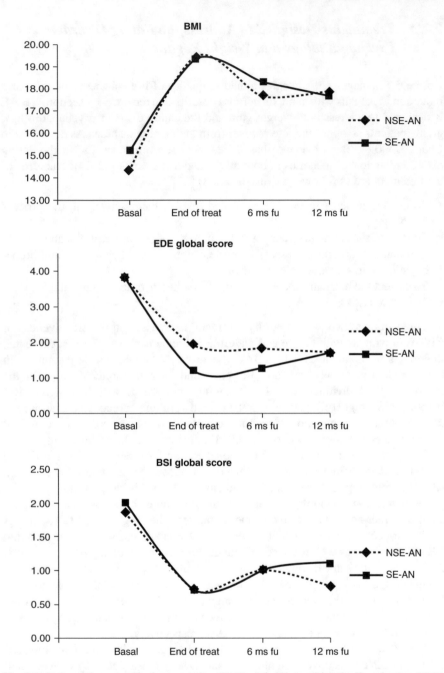

Fig. 9.1 Estimated means of body mass index (BMI), global Eating Disorder Examination (EDE) and Brief Symptom Inventory (BSI) scores from baseline to 12-month follow-up in patients with severe and enduring anorexia nervosa (SE-AN) and anorexia nervosa of less than 7 years' duration (NSE-AN). Estimates were obtained using mixed-effects models

From Calugi S, El Ghoch M, Dalle Grave R. Intensive enhanced cognitive behavioural therapy for severe and enduring anorexia nervosa: A longitudinal outcome study. Behav Res Ther. 2017;89:41–8. doi:10.1016/j.brat.2016.11.006. Reprinted with the permission of Elsevier nervosa and those with shorter-duration of the disorder displayed similar rates of good BMI outcome (40.7% and 44.0%, respectively) and full response (33.3% and 32.0%, respectively) at 12-month follow-up.

The third study, conducted by Raykos et al., assessed the effect of disorder severity or duration upon outpatient CBT-E outcomes in a sample of 134 patients with anorexia nervosa [10]. Although the results were limited by the high attrition at follow-up, neither disorder severity nor duration predicted end-of-treatment outcome, and, as in our research, patients with more severe or long-standing anorexia nervosa exhibited a similar degree of improvement as patients with anorexia nervosa of more recent onset [10].

These findings show that a large group of patients with severe and enduring anorexia nervosa can, in fact, be effectively treated via an evidence-based programme geared towards addressing weight regain and resolving the eating disorder psychopathology. They also underscore the importance of designing treatments that optimize patient engagement—a key feature of CBT-E. In fact, it is likely that the promising outcomes seen in the large subgroup of patients with severe and enduring anorexia nervosa treated with CBT-E may be partly due to the collaborative style of the treatment, which is focused on "empowering" rather than coercing patients, and includes specific procedures designed to prevent relapse [2]. Moreover, the CBT-E strategy of not broaching weight regain directly in Step One may also be a contributing factor (see Chap. 3). Indeed, it is our clinical experience that most patients, even those with severe and enduring anorexia nervosa, accept the goals of CBT-E Step One, namely to engage patients, help them understand the main mechanisms maintaining their eating disorder, explore the nature and outcome of prior treatments, and discuss the pros and cons of change and gaining weight, but not to begin the process of weight regain. If patients do not conclude that they need to address their low weight after 4–8 weeks, CBT-E is discontinued, but this seldom occurs, even in patients with severe and enduring anorexia nervosa.

9.3   A Pragmatic Clinical Approach to Managing Patients with Severe and Enduring Anorexia Nervosa

In our clinical practice, if a patient has severe and enduring anorexia nervosa, we dedicate one or two sessions after the initial assessment to discussing with them the pros and cons of embarking on a course of treatment like CBT-E which is focused on change, and ultimately weight regain, as opposed to one that prioritizes improving their quality of life and achieving medical stabilization over weight regain and recovery. We follow the usual approach in CBT-E, attempting to engage patients and educating them on the mechanisms maintaining their eating disorder, which from a CBT perspective are not appreciably different from those acting in patients with anorexia nervosa of shorter duration. We also stress that it is very difficult to maintain stable medical conditions if malnutrition is severe, and that the available data indicate that it is possible even after many years of illness to achieve a marked improvement, and in some cases remission. It is then up to the patient to decide how they want to proceed. In our experience, most choose to attempt change, and we therefore support their decision and enrol them on the appropriate programme. If, however, they do not yet feel ready for change, we help them manage their illness as best we can.

Vignette

The patient is a 30-year-old woman with severe and enduring anorexia nervosa. The onset of the eating disorder was at the age of 15 years, when she had a body weight of 70 kg (BMI 24.2), and embarked on a strict diet in order to lose weight. Over the first 6 months she lost weight rapidly, reaching as low as 43 kg (BMI 14.9), at which point she was admitted to a medical unit, where she was fed through a nasogastric tube in order to treat her severe malnutrition. After discharge she was referred to a specialist family-based outpatient treatment, which helped her to achieve a body weight of 58 kg (BMI 20.0) and resumption of regular periods.

However, at the age of 18 years, when she started university, she started rigorously dieting again, once again rapidly losing weight, which fell to 45 kg (BMI 15.6), prompting her admission to a specialist eclectic inpatient treatment for eating disorder. After 5 months, she was discharged with a body weight of 57.5 kg (BMI 19.9), but no mitigation of her preoccupation with shape and weight. By this time she had also been diagnosed with comorbid obsessive-compulsive disorder, for which she was prescribed a combination of antidepressant and neuroleptic agents. She was regularly seeing a psychologist, but rapidly lost the weight she had regained in the unit, and after 6 months was therefore re-hospitalized. She received another course of the same inpatient treatment for eating disorder, during which she regained weight but subsequently relapsed after discharge. This cycle of regain and relapse continued with another six inpatient admissions, which ultimately failed to achieve their long-term goals, despite the patient receiving psychological and psychopharmacological support in the interim.

When she was eventually referred to our unit, she had a body weight of 48 kg (BMI 16.9) and was amenorrhoeic. At the assessment and preparation session with our team, she reported that this body weight had remained stable over the previous 4 weeks, despite her following extreme and rigid dietary rules accompanied by frequent food checking (she weighed and counted the calories in all foods she was to eat), and excessive exercising (walking for about 2 h every day). She also reported extreme fear of weight gain, overvaluation of shape and weight, frequent body checking, feeling fat, mood swings, irritability, social withdrawal, and that she had been forced to take a leave of absence from work due to her difficulty in concentrating. Interestingly, bearing in mind her former diagnosis, the patient reported no obsessions or compulsions unrelated to food and eating.

The therapist discussed with the patient the relative pros and cons of undergoing a treatment, like CBT-E, designed to help her recover, or one focused on harm reduction and quality of life improvement. After having received detailed information about the two treatments, the patient decided to start CBT-E as she appreciated that there was a need for change. In particular, she was reassured that

Table 9.2 Changes in body weight, eating disorder and general psychopathology and clinical impairment scores in a patient with severe and enduring anorexia nervosa

	Before CBT-E	After CBT-E	20-week follow-up	60-week follow-up
Body weight (kg)	48	55	57	58
Body mass index (BMI)	16.9	19	19.7	20
Eating disorder examination questionnaire				
Dietary restraint	4.3	2.7	1.8	1.8
Eating concern	5.1	2.8	2.1	1.8
Weight concern	3.8	1.8	1.6	1.5
Shape concern	5.3	2.8	2.0	2.1
Global score	4.6	2.5	1.9	1.8
Clinical impairment assessment	32.6	15.4	10.3	5.6
Brief symptom inventory	2.1	0.8	0.6	0.6

CBT-E Enhanced cognitive behavioural therapy

goals of CBT-E Step One involved helping her understand the psychological processes maintaining her eating disorder, and weighing up the implications of addressing both the eating disorder psychopathology and regaining weight. This contrasted starkly with all her previous treatments, whose primary focus had been weight regain.

The patient progressed through Step One, albeit with a lot of effort, and after 4 weeks decided that she was ready to attempt to regain weight and address her eating disorder psychopathology. In Step Two, her attempts to regain weight were hampered by her excessive exercising and high number of dietary rules. However, by means of the CBT-E strategy designed to address her overvaluation of shape and weight and her dietary restraint and restriction in combination, she was able to achieve a body weight of 55 kg (BMI 19.0) and a reduction in eating disorder and general psychopathology and clinical impairment scores by the end of the treatment. Unlike on previous occasions, this improvement continued after the treatment ended, and at 60-week follow-up she had a body weight of 58 kg (BMI 20.0) and her eating disorder psychopathology remained in remission (Table 9.2).

References

1. Broomfield C, Stedal K, Touyz S, Rhodes P. Labeling and defining severe and enduring anorexia nervosa: a systematic review and critical analysis. Int J Eat Disord. 2017;50(6):611–23. https://doi.org/10.1002/eat.22715.
2. Dalle Grave R. Severe and enduring anorexia nervosa: no easy solutions. Int J Eat Disord. 2020;53:1320–1. https://doi.org/10.1002/eat.23295.
3. American Psychiatric Association. Diagnostic and statistical manual of mental disorders, (DSM-5). Arlington: American Psychiatric Publishing; 2013.

4. Button EJ, Chadalavada B, Palmer RL. Mortality and predictors of death in a cohort of patients presenting to an eating disorders service. Int J Eat Disord. 2010;43(5):387–92. https://doi.org/10.1002/eat.20715.

5. Dalle Grave R, Sartirana M, El Ghoch M, Calugi S. DSM-5 severity specifiers for anorexia nervosa and treatment outcomes in adult females. Eat Behav. 2018;31:18–23. https://doi.org/10.1016/j.eatbeh.2018.07.006.

6. Wonderlich SA, Bulik CM, Schmidt U, Steiger H, Hoek HW. Severe and enduring anorexia nervosa: update and observations about the current clinical reality. Int J Eat Disord. 2020;53(8):1303–12. https://doi.org/10.1002/eat.23283.

7. Steinhausen HC. The outcome of anorexia nervosa in the 20th century. Am J Psychiatry. 2002;159(8):1284–93. https://doi.org/10.1176/appi.ajp.159.8.1284.

8. Wild B, Friederich HC, Zipfel S, Resmark G, Giel K, Teufel M, et al. Predictors of outcomes in outpatients with anorexia nervosa—results from the ANTOP study. Psychiatry Res. 2016;244:45–50. https://doi.org/10.1016/j.psychres.2016.07.002.

9. Calugi S, El Ghoch M, Dalle Grave R. Intensive enhanced cognitive behavioural therapy for severe and enduring anorexia nervosa: a longitudinal outcome study. Behav Res Ther. 2017;89:41–8. https://doi.org/10.1016/j.brat.2016.11.006.

10. Raykos BC, Erceg-Hurn DM, McEvoy PM, Fursland A, Waller G. Severe and enduring anorexia nervosa? Illness severity and duration are unrelated to outcomes from cognitive behaviour therapy. J Consult Clin Psychol. 2018;86(8):702–9. https://doi.org/10.1037/ccp0000319.

11. Dobrescu SR, Dinkler L, Gillberg C, Råstam M, Gillberg C, Wentz E. Anorexia nervosa: 30-year outcome. Br J Psychiatry. 2020;216(2):97–104. https://doi.org/10.1192/bjp.2019.113.

12. Eddy KT, Tabri N, Thomas JJ, Murray HB, Keshaviah A, Hastings E, et al. Recovery from anorexia nervosa and bulimia nervosa at 22-year follow-up. J Clin Psychiatry. 2017;78(2):184–9. https://doi.org/10.4088/JCP.15m10393.

13. Hay P, Touyz S. Classification challenges in the field of eating disorders: can severe and enduring anorexia nervosa be better defined? J Eat Disord. 2018;6:41. https://doi.org/10.1186/s40337-018-0229-8.

14. Ruggeri M, Leese M, Thornicroft G, Bisoffi G, Tansella M. Definition and prevalence of severe and persistent mental illness. Br J Psychiatry. 2000;177:149–55. https://doi.org/10.1192/bjp.177.2.149.

15. Goldner E. Treatment refusal in anorexia nervosa. Int J Eat Disord. 1989;8(3):297–306. https://doi.org/10.1002/1098-108x(198905)8:3<297::aid-eat2260080305>3.0.co;2-h.

16. Robinson P. Severe and enduring eating disorders (SEED): management of complex presentation of anorexia and bulimia nervosa. Chichester: Wiley-Blackwell Press; 2009.

17. Strober M. Managing the chronic, treatment-resistant patient with anorexia nervosa. Int J Eat Disord. 2004;36(3):245–55. https://doi.org/10.1002/eat.20054.

18. Yager J. Patients with chronic recalcitrant eating disorders. In: Yager J, Gwirtsman H, Edelstein C, editors. Special problems in managing eating disorder. Washington, DC: American Psychiatric Press; 1992.

19. Wonderlich S, Mitchell JE, Crosby RD, Myers TC, Kadlec K, Lahaise K, et al. Minimizing and treating chronicity in the eating disorders: a clinical overview. Int J Eat Disord. 2012;45(4):467–75. https://doi.org/10.1002/eat.20978.

20. Touyz S, Le Grange D, Lacey H, Hay P, Smith R, Maguire S, et al. Treating severe and enduring anorexia nervosa: a randomized controlled trial. Psychol Med. 2013;43(12):2501–11. https://doi.org/10.1017/s0033291713000949.

21. Touyz S, Le Grange D, Lacey H, Hay P. Managing severe and enduring anorexia nervosa: a clinician's guide. New York, NY: Taylor & Francis; 2016.

22. National Guideline Alliance. Eating disorders: Recognition and treatment. London: National Institute for Health and Care Excellence (UK); 2017 May. (NICE Guideline, No. 69.) London 2017.

23. Dalle Grave R, Calugi S. Cognitive behavior therapy for adolescents with eating disorders. New York: Guilford Press; 2020.
24. Fairburn CG. Cognitive behavior therapy and eating disorders. New York: Guilford Press; 2008.
25. Calugi S, Dalle Grave R, Marchesini G. Longstanding underweight eating disorder: associated features and treatment outcome. Psychother Res. 2013;23(3):315–23. https://doi.org/10.108 0/10503307.2012.717308.

Appendix A: The Eating Problem Check List

What Is It, and How Should It Be Used?

The Eating Problem Check List (EPCL) is a 16-item self-report measure designed to assess eating disorder behaviours and psychopathology in patients with eating disorders, session-by-session. The 15 items cover the principal behaviours and attitudes of eating disorder psychopathology expressed over the preceding 7 days.

The EPCL is quick and easy to complete, and therefore readily lends itself to integration into routine clinical practice in order to enable assessment of weekly changes. The tool allows the clinician and the patient to assess, through the review of each single item score, the change occurring in specific eating disorder psychopathology expressions at weekly intervals. Moreover, through the two subscale scores (i.e., Body Image and Eating Concerns), the tool permits assessment of weekly changes in the core psychopathology of eating disorders. As an aid for clinicians and patients in identifying areas of improvement and/or deterioration, the EPCL enables prompt focusing of the treatment on specific expressions of an individual's eating disorder psychopathology. Moreover, it enables the detection of sudden gains (i.e. large, rapid and stable changes in symptomatology between two consecutive treatment sessions), which seem to be associated with greater overall post-treatment symptom reduction and better outcomes. In addition, associations between sudden gains and short- and long-term improvements also appear to have a positive impact on therapeutic alliance.

In our clinical practice, we find it very useful to carefully review and discuss with the patient the EPCL single item scores on a weekly basis (after the CBT-E collaborative weighing procedure). Indeed, weekly review of the EPCL, in conjunction with the self-monitoring records review, helps to highlight the changes that patients have made (when there is a weekly change of at least one point in one or more EPCL items), and identify the behavioural expressions of their eating disorder psychopathology that remain to be addressed by the treatment. What is more, by recording weekly EPCL data on a spreadsheet, it is possible to observe whether—as

© The Author(s), under exclusive license to Springer Nature
Switzerland AG 2021
R. Dalle Grave et al., *Complex Cases and Comorbidity in Eating Disorders*,
https://doi.org/10.1007/978-3-030-69341-1

assumed by CBT-E theory—modification of certain behaviours (e.g. adopting regular eating, reducing dietary restraint, weekly weighing, and/or interrupting dysfunctional body checking) is in fact associated with a reduction in concerns about eating, shape and weight over time—one of the primary goals of CBT-E.

Status of the EPCL

The design and validation of the EPCL has been published in the journal *Eating Disorders* [1]. The EPCL has demonstrated good internal consistency, test–retest reliability and concurrent and criterion validity, and principal component analysis of the session-by-session data identified two factors ("eating concerns" and "body image concerns") that accounted for 51.3% of the variance. Session-by-session analysis has indicated that the EPCL is able to identify weekly specific changes and/ or deterioration in eating disorder psychopathology.

Scoring the EPCL

The total score is obtained by adding scores for the items in Section Two, while scores for the two subscales are given by the sum of the following items, also in the second section: Body Image Concern, the sum of the scores for items 4, 5, 6, 7 and 8; Eating Concern, the sum of the scores for items 1, 2, 3 and 9.

Copyright

The EPCL is freely available for non-for-profit research, and no permission need be sought for non-commercial research use. For commercial use of the EPCL, contact: rdalleg@tin.it

Reference
1. Dalle Grave R, Sartirana M, Milanese C, El Ghoch M, Brocco C, Pellicone C, et al. Validity and reliability of the Eating Problem Checklist. Eat Disord. 2019;27(4):384–99. doi:10.1080/10640266.2018.1528084.

The Eating Problem Checklist (EPCL) 3.1

INSTRUCTIONS: The following questions are about the past 7 days only. Please read each question carefully. Please answer all the questions so that they are true for you. Thank you.

In the past 7 days, how often *(indicate the number of times that this has occurred in the box on the right)*	**No. of episodes**
… have you eaten a large amount of food with a sense of having lost control (i.e. an objective binge-eating episode)?	
… have you eaten a not large amount of food with a sense of having lost control (i.e. a subjective binge-eating episode)?	
… have you made yourself sick (vomited) as a means of controlling your shape and weight?	
… have you taken laxatives as a means of controlling your shape and weight?	
… have you taken diuretics (water pills) as a means of controlling your shape and weight?	
… have you exercised excessively as a means of controlling your weight, shape or amount of fat, or to burn extra calories?	
… have you weighed yourself?	

In the past 7 days, how often *(tick which box is true for you)*	**0** **Never**	**1** **Rarely**	**2** **Sometimes**	**3** **Often**	**4** **Always**
1. … have you avoided some foods as a means of controlling your weight, shape and/or eating?					
2. … have you reduced your food portions as a means of controlling your weight, shape and/or eating?					
3. … have you checked your food (e.g. calorie counting, weighing food, checking the food's nutritional content)?					
4. … have you checked your shape (e.g. looking at parts of your body in the mirror, measuring the circumference of parts of your body, or compared your body shape with that of other people)?					
5. … have you avoided your body (e.g. avoided weighing, avoided particular clothes, avoided looking at my body)?					
6. … have you felt fat?					
7. … have you been worried about your weight?					
8. … have you been worried about your shape?					
9. … have you been worried about your eating control?					

How many "days of change" have you had?
N.B.: A day of change is when you did your best to change using the procedures you have learned during treatment

Eating Problem Checklist (EPCL) Weekly Changes Summary Spreadsheet

Data																			
Week																			
Body weight (kg)																			
Objective binge eating[a]																			
Subjective binge eating[a]																			
Vomiting[a]																			
Laxatives[a]																			
Diuretics[a]																			
Excessive exercising[a]																			
Weight checking[a]																			
Food avoidance[b]																			
Reduction of food portions[b]																			
Food checking[b]																			
Body shape checking[b]																			
Body avoidance[b]																			
Feeling fat[b]																			
Weight concern[b]																			
Body shape concern[b]																			
Eating concern[b]																			

[a]Number of events in the last 7 days
[b]Never = 0, rarely = 1, sometimes = 2, often = 3 and always = 4

Appendix B: The Starvation Symptom Inventory

What Is It, and How Should It Be Used?

The Starvation Symptoms Inventory (SSI) is a 15-item self-report measure that examines the symptoms of starvation in underweight patients with eating disorders. It is focused on the past 28 days. The SSI can be easily integrated into routine clinical practice as a means of assessing starvation symptoms in underweight patients with eating disorders, and how they evolve during the process of weight restoration in those who attend specialized eating disorder treatments. It can be also used in research evaluating the effects of eating disorder treatments.

Status of the SSI

The design and validation of the SSI has been published in the journal *Nutrients* [1]. Principal component analysis identified a single-factor, 15-item scale which demonstrated good internal consistency (alpha = 0.91) and test–retest reliability ($r = 0.90$). The SSI global score was significantly correlated with eating disorder and general psychopathology scores, demonstrating good convergent validity. SSI scores were significantly higher in the anorexia nervosa sample than in healthy control, not-underweight eating disorder, and bipolar/depressive episode samples. These findings suggest that the SSI is a valid self-report questionnaire that may provide important clinical information regarding symptoms of starvation in patients with anorexia nervosa.

The structure of the SSI mirrors that of the EDE-Q, and participants are asked to provide an estimate of the number of days out of the preceding 28 (4 weeks) in which they have experienced each symptom on a 7-point Likert scale ranging from "never" (0) to "always" (6).

R. Dalle Grave et al., *Complex Cases and Comorbidity in Eating Disorders*, https://doi.org/10.1007/978-3-030-69341-1

Scoring the SSI

The global SSI score is obtained by adding the scores for the 15 items in the questionnaire. The resulting scores range from 0 to 90, with the highest scores indicating greater frequency of starvation symptoms experienced over the preceding 28 days. In patients with anorexia nervosa the average score obtained is 55.1, while healthy controls score an average of 10.4.

Copyright

The SSI (and its items) is freely available for not-for-profit research, and no permission need be sought for non-commercial research. For commercial use of the SSI, contact: rdalleg@tin.it

Reference
1. Calugi S, Miniati M, Milanese C, Sartirana M, El Ghoch M, Dalle Grave R. The Starvation Symptom Inventory: development and psychometric properties. Nutrients. 2017;9(9):967. doi:10.3390/nu9090967

The Starvation Symptom Inventory (SSI)

INSTRUCTIONS: The following questions are about the past 4 weeks *(28 days)*. Please read each question carefully and respond to ALL questions. Thank you.

How many times in the last 28 days have you:	Never	1–5 days	6–12 days	13–15 days	16–22 days	23–27 days	Every day
Worried about food?							
Collected recipes, menus or cookbooks?							
Increased your consumption of tea, coffee or spices?							
Felt depressed?							
Felt anxious?							
Felt irritable?							
Had mood swings (between excitement and depression)?							
Stayed away from other people?							

Experienced a loss of concentration?							
Felt apathetic?							
Had disturbed sleep?							
Felt weak?							
Experienced a lack of interest in sex?							
Felt cold?							
Felt full early?							

Printed in the United States
by Baker & Taylor Publisher Services